OXFORD MEDICAL P[...]

Fighting for Life

Fighting for Life

*An introduction to the
Intensive Care Unit*

Gilbert Park
and
Kieron Saunders

Oxford   New York   Melbourne
OXFORD UNIVERSITY PRESS
1996

Oxford University Press, Walton Street, Oxford OX2 6DR

Oxford   New York
Athens   Auckland   Bangkok   Bombay
Calcutta   Cape Town   Dar es Salaam   Delhi
Florence   Hong Kong   Istanbul   Karachi
Kuala Lumpur   Madras   Madrid   Melbourne
Mexico City   Nairobi   Paris   Singapore
Taipei   Tokyo   Toronto

and associated companies in
Berlin   Ibadan

Oxford is a trade mark of Oxford University Press

Published in the United States
by Oxford University Press Inc., New York

A catalogue record for this book is available from the British Library

Library of Congress Cataloging in Publication Data
(Data available)

ISBN 0 19 262582 9 hb
ISBN 0 19 262572 1 pbk

Typeset by EXPO Holdings, Malaysia

Printed in Great Britain by
Biddles Ltd, Guildford

To Jay and Pascale
for their typing and drawing
and so much more

Foreword

P. G. M. Wallace
President, Intensive Care Society

The general public's perception of Intensive Care is largely gleaned from medical soap operas on TV. When the reality of critical illness is faced as patient or relative the circumstances and surroundings are complicated, confusing, and often frightening to the layman. However much time and care is taken by medical staff in explanation, it is difficult for stunned and anxious relatives to comprehend all details described to them. It is here that this little book has a unique contribution to make in expanding the understanding of Intensive Care. While never substituting for personal communication, this book will permit a fuller understanding of the surroundings and the medical conditions involved in Intensive Care and the treatment being undertaken. Written in plain language it will allow the layman to absorb information at his or her own rate, in their own time and not only supplement doctors' and nurses' explanations but suggest relevant questions that may be asked.

I compliment the authors on their success in covering so many aspects of Intensive Care in approximately 100 pages. Questions we are asked as Intensive Care doctors are clearly explained and I am sure that relatives and, indeed, many patients will appreciate the opportunity to gain a deeper understanding of the unfortunate circumstances in which they find themselves. In my opinion a book with a chapter entitled 'Feelings' has the right priorities especially when coupled with clear explanation of the technical side of Intensive Care on which we too often concentrate.

I commend the authors on their initiative and am certain that all involved in Intensive Care, whether staff, patients, or relatives will find this a most useful publication.

Preface

'Fighting for life' is a phrase frequently used by the media to describe simply the battle for survival of a seriously ill or injured person in an intensive care unit (ICU). It aptly describes the predicament in which the unfortunate patient finds themselves, as well as the work of all those employed in intensive care. This book *Fighting for life* is a simple guide to some of the more serious conditions which bring patients to intensive care, how they are then cared for, the techniques, drugs, and machines that are used in that care, and most important of all, the people who carry out that care.

Many doctors realized from the frequent questions asked by patients, and their relatives and friends, that there was a real need for a simple guide in layman's language. This book necessarily contains some medical and technical terms, but all are clearly and simply explained. To achieve this aim needed two types of expertise: a medical man with an intimate knowledge and experience of intensive care and a Fleet Street journalist to turn that vast wealth of medical detail into everyday words.

Sometimes specialist phrases and words often used in intensive care units have been included, so that readers will recognize the words used in these units. Most of the words are pronounced exactly as they look, saying every letter. For those that are not, we give a guide to pronunciation.

The style is simple, but we hope informative. It is difficult to be lighthearted in any way about something so serious as fighting for life. There is humour in intensive care units, but some of it tends to be 'black' and is used as a safety valve for staff. It is difficult to record that in the sterile pages of a book without causing offence.

This book is concise – but it took many hours of debate to distil the kind of information that could fill an encyclopedia – and gallons of late-night coffee. It is not intended to be a comprehensive medical tome, or a detailed nursing guide. The idea for the book came from the Association of Anaesthetists and the Intensive Care Society of Great Britain and Northern Ireland, representing many of the doctors in Great Britain who care for the critically ill. We are grateful to them for allowing us to use this idea and for their support.

If you have bought this book because you, or a member of your family or a friend, are receiving treatment in an intensive care unit and, after reading it, you still have out-standing questions, never be afraid to ask the ICU staff. They will be only too happy to explain.

We are grateful to many people who have patiently read early versions of this book and made many helpful sugges-tions including: Giles Morgan (Truro Hospital); Fulton Gillespie (*Cambridge Evening News*); Barry Brignell (Brignells Bookbinders); William Macrae (Association of Anaesthetists); and the staff of Oxford University Press.

Finally, each of the authors has paraphrased a quotation that has guided them through the preparation of this book.

Gilbert Park:

> 'Don't make the remedy worse than the disease'.
> *Francis Bacon, English Lord Chancellor 1561–1626.*

Kieron Saunders:

> 'There is no fear worse than the fear of the unknown'.
> *Captain James T. Kirk of the Starship Enterprise.*

Cambridge	G. P.
London	K. S.
May 1995	

Contents

1

History

Intensive care started with Florence Nightingale during the Crimean War. She first suggested grouping together all the very seriously ill patients in one place.

Most patients in any intensive care unit have a serious or life-threatening problem. Today, different types of intensive care units have developed for patients suffering an enormous variety of ailments.

Many intensive care units have a large number of patients who cannot breathe unaided and usually have problems associated with their heart or the major blood vessels.

The modern history of intensive care really began in the 1950s with the polio epidemic in Scandinavia, which also spread to Great Britain. Polio attacks the nerves supplying the muscles and its victims die because they cannot breathe. Scandinavian doctors found they could save large numbers of patients by artificially aiding their breathing. They did this by hand, using rubber bags which they squeezed to push air into the lungs. Then a machine was devised to carry on this breathing mechanically. This was the first 'iron lung'.

It was then realized that many other people who died from breathing problems after operations could be saved if a machine took over their breathing. Surgical patients suffering breathing troubles, because of the effects of disease or drugs, were then put on breathing machines for some time until they recovered and were able to breathe unaided.

Before legislation in the United Kingdom enforced the widespread use of seat-belts many victims of road crashes died from chest injuries. Breaking six or more ribs would prove fatal because it had a disastrous effect on the working of the lungs. Putting the victim on a ventilator to restore normal chest and lung function until the ribs repaired saved hundred of lives. From this modest beginning today's varied and highly complex intensive care units with all their hi-tec machines and sophisticated drugs developed.

Today's intensive care units (ICUs) treat patients whose many vital bodily functions have failed at the same time, not just the lungs. Patients with single-organ failure will now stay in an intensive care unit for only a few days.

Because we will discuss the various organs found in the body, we have included a diagram showing some of them. More detailed diagrams are included in appropriate places.

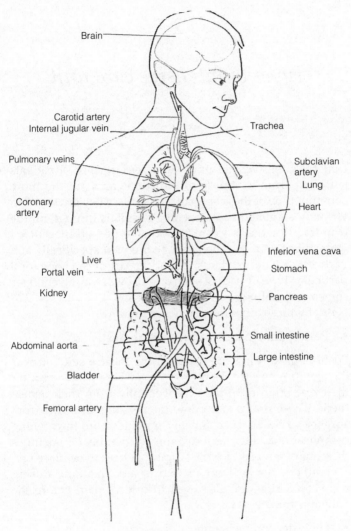

Some parts of the body.

2

Types of intensive care unit

General intensive care units cater for critically ill patients suffering from a variety of afflictions and are the more common type of these specialized wards. They are found in virtually all general and teaching hospitals throughout the country. But there are many other types of specialized intensive care units. These can be targeted specifically at a particular injury or illness, a specific part of the body, or a particular type of patient such as a baby or young child, or someone simply recovering from surgery.

Briefly these other intensive care units are:

- Post-operative units or recovery rooms

Post-operative units are found in the theatre suite or near an operating theatre. They are rooms where people go after their operation until they recover fully from their anaesthetic. These rooms also allow the person recovering from surgery to be watched for any imminent life-threatening complications, such as breathing difficulties. Sometimes there may be a need for the surgical patient to be placed on a ventilator for an hour or two to aid breathing during recovery. Drugs are also used to control pain before the patient is transferred to a ward.

- High-dependency units

A high-dependency unit is midway between a full intensive care unit and a ward. It is a place where patients needing close monitoring, or specific treatment, can be catered for rather than on a ward where there may be an insufficient number of nurses available for the amount of surveillance or treatment required. The high dependency unit will, for example, allow patients suffering from diabetes to have their blood levels of glucose and insulin kept under close control. In a similar way to the recovery room, patients recovering from surgery can also have drug infusions to control the pain of their operation.

A high-dependency unit can also be used as a 'half-way house' from the full intensive care unit before the patient moves on to a general ward.

• Coronary care units

Most large district general hospitals have a coronary care unit which caters solely for people who have suffered heart attacks. These people need special monitoring and a nurse in close attendance watching for any signs of irregularity of the heartbeat (arrhythmia). Heart-attack victims can often suffer heart failure, or the heart just stops because of an arrhythmia, and they need immediate attention. Heart failure is caused by a liquid build-up in the tissue of the lungs (pulmonary oedema). (This is different from pneumonia, when there is infection in the air sacs in the lungs.)

The coronary care unit has machines to infuse the drugs necessary to try and prevent these conditions and electrical stimulation or pacemakers to maintain a normal heart rate.

• Paediatric intensive care units

These units are referred to commonly as PICUs. Sick children tend to thrive better when grouped together with patients of their own age. They can be badly affected by the suffering of elderly patients. There are also particular problems in dealing with very ill children because of their size, which means that smaller equipment and different nursing skills are needed.

Paediatric intensive care units tend to be lighter and brighter places with much more gaudy decoration than a general intensive care unit. There is also a much more relaxed and noisy atmosphere in these units and the nurses tend to be more casually dressed.

Children in PICUs are usually recovering from operations or infections such as croup, meningitis, and epiglottitis, or have been injured in an accident. Fortunately, children heal faster than adults and their stay in such units is often much shorter.

PICUs tend to be available only in large teaching hospitals. In district general hospitals critically ill children are treated in general ICUs alongside adults, usually with good results. If they have special needs then these children will be transferred to a PICU.

- Neonatal intensive care units or special care baby units

These units also have an abbreviated name and are universally known as SCBUs (pronounced 'skiboos'). They cater for newborn and premature babies who have problems at birth. Others are recovering from surgical operations or have some illness such as pneumonia.

- Neuro-intensive care units

Neuro-intensive care units are normally found only in a large regional or teaching hospital where the specialized expertise required for this type of care is concentrated. The neuro units are sometimes divided into 'neurosurgical' for those recovering from lengthy brain operations and 'neuro-trauma' for the treatment of people who have had serious head injuries from accidents such as road crashes.

- Cardiac surgery intensive care units

These units are used for patients recovering after serious heart operations and other big chest operations.

- Renal intensive care units

Usually there is only one renal intensive care unit serving each region of the country. People with kidney failure occasionally need breathing machines but they do need dialysis. These units cater for that.

- Liver intensive care units

There are only a few of these throughout the country. They deal with patients with liver failure and the associated liver transplant programme.

- Burns intensive care units

These again tend to be limited to one per region and, as the name implies, cater specifically for serious burns patients.

- Poison intensive care units

There are only a few of these throughout the country. They are specifically designed to cater for those people who suffer from deliberate self-poisoning or accidental self-poisoning. Accidental self-poisonings tend to be the victims of industrial or farming accidents.

- Spinal injury units

These are specialist units dealing only with the aftercare of patients who have suffered damage to their neck or other part of the spinal cord. A few of these patients will need help with their breathing.

3

People

The patient fighting for life needs the help of a huge, dedicated, and highly skilled team. A critically ill person is virtually incapable of doing anything for themselves and in most cases is even more helpless than a healthy new born baby. An intensive care unit does not repair or cure the seriously ill. Its job is to keep the patient alive while specialists, often drawn from other departments in the hospital, organize the treatments that will eventually lead to recovery. That may sound simple, but it is not.

The successful intensive care unit requires a team of highly qualified, well organized, and well disciplined medical, nursing, and support staff. They must be capable of communicating swiftly and easily with each other and liaising and communicating with an enormous network of other specialists. These include the medical, nursing, paramedic, and ancillary staff throughout the hospital on whose resources they must call daily.

Many large hospitals are linked to the medical departments of a university. Senior medical people working in an intensive care unit may also work in a university medical department carrying out vital research, training, and other work. For this reason, a consultant – for example – may also have the title of Professor.

In Britain each intensive care unit is run by a director or consultant in charge. He or she will be a senior consultant trained in the care of the critically ill. In Britain 80% of the members of the Intensive Care Society are anaesthetists. This is because intensive care grew from the need to assist the breathing of critically ill patients, which is the expertise of anaesthetists. Elsewhere in the world doctors from other specialties, such as medicine, commonly run the intensive care unit.

The director is directly responsible in all medical matters to the medical director of the hospital. On other administrative and managerial matters he reports to the hospital's chief executive. The director's wide range of duties include monitoring and advising on the care of the patients in the unit and researching and improving drugs, machines, and many aspects of intensive care.

The director will represent the unit at meetings in the hospital and locally, as well as at specialist conferences, seminars, and other meetings at home and abroad. The director operates very much as the managing director of a company while still being heavily involved in the day-to-day work on the 'shop floor'. The director, like all the medical and nursing staff, is on call for emergencies.

The director is always keen to meet relatives of the patients admitted to the unit and deal with problems which cannot be sorted out by other members of the team. However, the director is a busy person and cannot always see relatives instantly.

Consultants

Working alongside the director will be other consultants. They are each experts in their field and make their own decisions about patient care in consultation with their colleagues and experts in other hospital departments. One consultant is always on call 24 hours a day, in each unit.

Trainee Doctors

Working under the supervision of consultants will be trainee doctors. These are fully qualified doctors working their way up the promotional ladder towards consultant status. They may be training to eventually work in an intensive care unit themselves, but most are learning about the intensive care of the critically ill as part of their general training towards some other specialized area of medicine.

Consultants and trainees make several ward rounds each day in the unit to monitor the care and progress of their patients. On normal medical wards there is usually only one ward round a day, but the special conditions and the critical state of the patients in intensive care require more frequent monitoring.

The chart over the page shows the hierarchy of doctors in a hospital.

In large teaching hospitals in major cities across Britain and Ireland there will be a number of specialized intensive care units in addition to the general intensive care unit (see Chapter 2, Types of intensive care unit). These special departments have different staffing arrangements and cater specifically for head injuries, heart surgery, critically ill children, kidney and liver patients, and occasionally poison victims.

Manager

At the director's right hand is the intensive care unit manager. The manager can be nursing qualified, or can be a trained manager from industry or other walk of life. The manager shoulders the administrative burden of the unit. The manager is responsible for the recruitment of nurses and ancillary workers and organizes their work rota, hours,

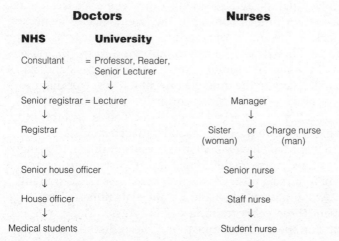

Doctors **Nurses**

NHS	**University**			
Consultant	= Professor, Reader, Senior Lecturer			
↓	↓			
Senior registrar = Lecturer			Manager	
↓			↓	
Registrar			Sister (woman)	or Charge nurse (man)
↓			↓	
Senior house officer			Senior nurse	
↓			↓	
House officer			Staff nurse	
↓			↓	
Medical students			Student nurse	

Medical and nursing hierarchy. You may meet students in the intensive care unit but they do not treat patients.

holidays, and training. The manager is also responsible for the discipline of all non-medical staff.

Ward clerk

The manager and other unit workers are assisted in the ward by the ward clerk. The ward clerk acts as the unit receptionist and carries out some secretarial duties including maintaining patient records.

Nurses

Nurses play a major part in the practical care of the critically ill. There will be up to seven nurses allocated on rota to each patient in intensive care because the work is so labour intensive. Some very sick patients, particularly those on ventilators and receiving other complex treatments, need two nurses constantly in attendance. The nurses' work on the unit is organized by the senior sister or charge nurse. They delegate responsibility in turn to other sisters in the unit. The senior sister maintains the standard of nursing care in the unit, ensures nurses are working properly, and are being trained correctly.

The senior sister or charge nurse liaises with all other departments in the hospital and patients' families.

Sisters will have spent three years training to achieve registered nurse qualifications and at least a fourth year in a senior nursing post, followed by three years' ICU training.

At the patient's bedside are the staff nurses. They have spent three years training to be a nurse. Many will also have a specialist qualification. These dedicated workers carry out the 24-hour specialized care of the patients on the unit. They regularly check the vast and complex array of machines that keep the patients alive and administer the individual treatment each patient requires. They move, feed, and clean their seriously ill patients and do everything their patients cannot do for themselves. Nurses are the unit workers who have the most contact with patients, their relatives, their friends, and other visitors. They can naturally become very emotionally involved in their patients' fight for life.

Nurses are in turn assisted by nursing auxiliaries. They are not qualified nurses but carry out work assigned to them by nurses. They also have to be sympathetic, caring people.

Paramedical staff

Working closely with the nurses and medical staff are the paramedical staff. These are drawn from other hospital departments such as physiotherapy, speech and language therapy, X-ray, cardiography, pharmacy and dietetics.

4

Shock

Shock is a killer. It can be caused by an accident which brings on sudden blood or fluid loss, or heart failure, infection, or allergy. Shock is a failure of the body to supply the cells with nutrients, mainly oxygen, and remove waste material. Doctors and nurses recognize it first by seeing their patient looking extremely ill. An immediate check on blood pressure will usually confirm this by showing it to be low.

Blood pressure is caused by the heart pumping blood around the body against the resistance of the blood vessels, which is affected partly by their size. The less the heart works, the lower the pressure in the arteries.

Blood vessels react to the output of the heart and dilate or contract to keep blood pressure stable in the body. Shock can be caused by the blood vessels opening wide (dilating) with a large flow of blood, but little pressure. As a result of shock essential organs such as the brain, heart, and kidney may not get sufficient oxygen for them to carry on working properly.

The heart is made mainly of muscle. Its ability to pump blood properly relies on the amount of blood returning to it, an efficient heart rate, and good, functioning muscles. If too little blood arrives the blood pressure will be low. Alternatively, too much blood arriving can cause the heart muscle to be stretched so that it cannot pump properly and again low blood pressure will result.

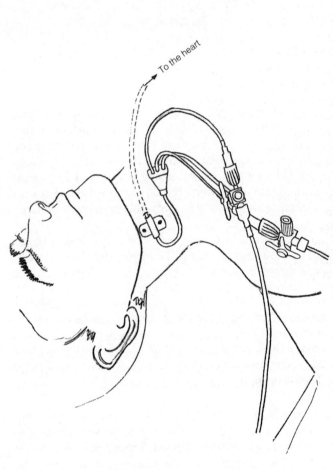

To the heart

Central venous catheter: a small tube used to measure the pressure of blood in the heart and to give drugs.

To measure the pressure of blood arriving back at the heart a thin tube, a central venous pressure line (CVP), is usually inserted into one of the veins near the heart by a doctor (see diagram opposite). It is linked to a measuring device known as a pressure transducer. This will give a visual display of the varying pressure at each beat of the heart.

Doctors will also need to find out if low blood pressure is caused by some damage or poisoning affecting the heart. This is done by using another sophisticated measuring device called a flow-directed pulmonary artery catheter, a Swan–Ganz® catheter. The Swan–Ganz catheter is fully explained in (Chapter 13, Equipment).

Output from the heart can also be affected by the speed at which it pumps. A very slow heartbeat means the heart is pumping slowly and not forcing much blood into the system. This will cause low blood pressure. A very fast beat can also cause low pressure because the heart does not have time to fill properly before the pumping action starts again. This usually happens when the heart rate reaches 160 beats per minute or more.

When treating all forms of shock the aims are the same:

- restore oxygen to the body's cells
- restore a proper blood volume with a transfusion if necessary
- ensure the heart is pumping at the right rate and power by correcting any abnormalities caused by poison, disease or injury.

Hypovolaemic shock

This is caused by a sudden loss of blood or fluid, such as in a serious injury in a road accident, or as a result of surgery or severe burning. It can also be the result of severe diarrhoea, diabetes, or peritonitis. If there is a sudden loss of blood then the shock is simply caused by not enough blood reaching the heart for it to pump. Hypovolaemia can also be caused by the sudden loss of fluid from the body — such as diarrhoea. This is because fluids flow from the blood to replace those lost elsewhere in the body. The treatment is to replace the fluid loss with either blood, plasma, or saline (salt and water). All are usually given directly into the veins in an intensive care unit. Plasma is part of the blood and is made up of proteins, salt, and water.

Cardiogenic shock

This happens when the heart muscle is damaged, as in a heart attack, or poisoned, such as in severe infection. The first treatment is to control the heart rate, which may be abnormal. This is done by drugs or electric stimulation. An electric shock can be given to the heart from outside the body to try and shock the heart back into line. The patient may need to be anaesthetized for this form of electrical treatment. It is usually used in cases of a high rate (ventricular fibrillation or ventricular tachycardia). When the heart rate is low (bradycardia) it is possible to insert a thin wire into the heart, through a vein in the neck, and control the heart by electrical impulses (pacemaker). If the heart is not pumping properly because it has been poisoned, or after a heart attack, then a variety of drugs can be used and these are called inotropes (described in detail in Chapter 15, Drugs).

Septic shock

This is a complex form of shock and may involve all the forms of treatment previously listed for shock. It is usually caused by toxins being released by bacteria, as a result of infection, but there are times when the source of the infection cannot be found. One of the problems septic shock causes is tiny blood vessels linking veins and arteries (capillaries) start to leak. Instead of the plasma staying in the capillaries it leaks to surrounding tissues. This has to be replaced artificially as with hypovolaemic shock. Another thing that may happen during septic shock is that the blood vessels all dilate. This causes a low blood pressure. The heart then pumps more blood into the system in a bid to compensate. To correct this drugs may be used to 'tighten up' the circulation. These are called vasoconstrictor drugs (see Chapter 15, Drugs).

In extreme forms of sepsis the heart does not pump well and cannot compensate. The blood vessels react by constricting. A drug may be used to open up the blood vessels again, called a vasodilator drug (see Chapter 15, Drugs).

Anaphylactic shock

(Pronounced 'ana-fil-actic'.) This is caused by an allergic reaction to a drug, bee sting, or some other substance. Shock occurs because the allergic reaction makes capillaries leak fluid and blood vessels dilate. The allergic reaction also causes wheeziness in the lungs, like asthma, and blotches to appear on the skin, like big blisters — known as skin wheals.

The treatment is to give oxygen, fluid intravenously, and adrenaline. The adrenaline stops the release of the substance causing this shock. It also opens up the lungs again and stops the wheeziness. Vasoconstrictor drugs can also be given to stop the dilation of the blood vessels.

5

Breathing difficulties

One of the reasons why people come into general intensive care units is because they have breathing problems and need help with their breathing, usually with a ventilator. Patients needing a ventilator may have stopped breathing and need the machine to take over the working of their lungs, or they may have severe breathing problems and need assistance. Breathing, although it may appear obvious, is essential for life. Breathing brings oxygen into the body and expels waste air, including carbon dioxide.

Conditions that may need the patient to go into an intensive care unit for help with breathing are:

- infections, such as pneumonia
- an operation, because of the effects of surgery, pain, cold, anaesthetic drugs, and a large blood transfusion
- severe asthma
- acute, or chronic, respiratory disease, such as bronchitis or emphysema
- chest injury or major chest operation
- heart failure
- the effects of drowning, smoke inhalation, or poisoning
- acute respiratory distress syndrome (ARDS), which can be the result of injury or disease elsewhere in the body, causing poisons to affect the lungs.

If it is at all possible, doctors will try to keep patients with breathing problems off a ventilator. Recovery may be quicker if a patient can carry on breathing naturally and fewer drugs are necessary in their treatment. To try and assist these patients, an oxygen face mask may be used. This simply increases the oxygen supply to the lungs. If there is lots of water in the lungs doctors may give the patient a diuretic (see Chapter 15, Drugs). This is a drug that increases the amount of urine passed by the body and drains fluids from the body. Patients wheezing from water in the lungs, or asthma, can also be given a drug that eases breathing called a bronchodilator (see Chapter 15, Drugs). This opens the tubes leading to the lungs.

The doctors can, in certain cases, also try a tight-fitting face mask which is something like a pilot's oxygen mask. This is known as a constant positive airways pressure mask (CPAP). It forces oxygen-enriched air at a minimum set pressure into the lungs so that they only partially collapse. It can also open up areas of the lungs that may have already collapsed.

If, however, none of these treatments improve the patients breathing they must be aided by a ventilator. A ventilator can simply be a pump that pushes in a preset quantity of oxygen and air a set number of times per minute. This is known as continuous mandatory ventilation (CMV) or intermittent positive pressure ventilation (IPPV). To do this the patient has to be heavily sedated or paralysed, because trying to breathe against the machine can cause a dangerously high pressure to build up in the lungs, which could burst them.

Nowadays 'triggers' can be built into the ventilator so that the patient sets their own breathing rate. The trigger senses when the patient is starting to breathe in and will cause the ventilator to operate. It is possible to alternate the patients own breathing through the machine with breathing set by the machine. This is known as synchronized intermittent mandatory ventilation (SIMV). This particular form of ventilation can be used to wean patients off a ventilator.

The use by the patients of their own lungs maintains muscle strength in the ribcage. Respiratory muscles, like any other muscle in the body, can waste without use. It is possible to gradually reduce the amount of machine breathing and increase the patient's own breaths. Also, as part of the weaning process, it is possible for the machine to support each breath by the patient. This simply lets the machine 'top up' each breath and is known as pressure support (ASB-assisted spontaneous breathing).

Another method of assistance is positive end expiratory pressure (PEEP). This keeps a certain level of pressure in the lungs as the patient breathes out so that the lungs do not partially collapse.

To support breathing for a short period you can use a face mask. For a longer period of breathing support it is quite common for people to have a tube inserted into their windpipe (trachea) to administer the gas mixture necessary for their breathing. This is what the staff refer to as intubation, or to intubate a patient.

The tube can take several routes (see diagram opposite). Through the mouth is one obvious one, but it is difficult to keep in place, although it can be tied or taped in. Movement of this tube could also damage the voice box (larynx). Ideally this route is not used for more than 10 days. Instead it is more common to use the nose (nasotracheal tube) or the neck by making a little hole and putting the tube in. This is known as a tracheostomy.

The problem with bypassing a natural airway is that it can increase the risk of infection – the nose usually filters and warms air entering the body. The gases being supplied artificially are completely dry and at room temperature. In that form they can damage the lining of the windpipe and the little tubes in the lungs. So, the gases have to be

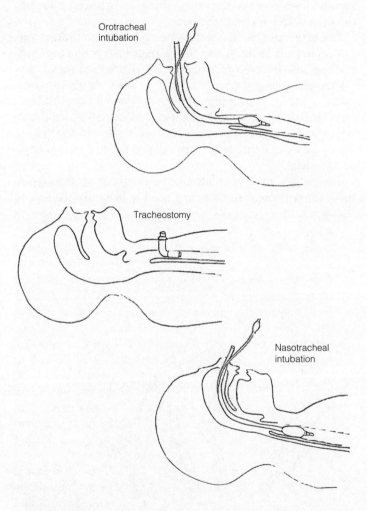

Tracheostomy tube: a breathing tube inserted into the windpipe through a small hole made in the neck. Also shown are tubes being put through the mouth and nose (orotracheal and nasotracheal intubation).

warmed and moistened before being received by the patient. This can be done by putting an artificial nose on the tube before it enters the body.

The artificial nose has a paper or plastic membrane over which the air leaving the lungs passes, condensing and leaving little droplets of moisture which are then picked up by the incoming dry gases. This is a recycling process. Some of these have an inbuilt filter to take out harmful bacteria. If it is necessary to moisten the air still more a hot water humidifier can be used instead of the artificial nose. The gases pass through warm water or across a warm, damp surface.

The patient on a ventilator, or being given air through a tube, cannot cough so there is a need to bring up the secre-

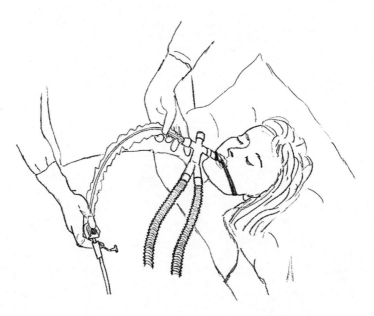

Suction tube, used to suck secretions from the lung.

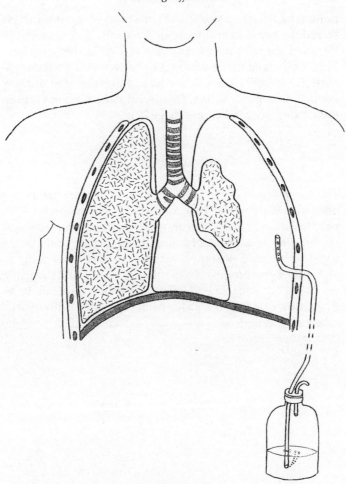

Chest tube, used to drain air and fluid from around the lung.

tions which form naturally. There may be more of those secretions because of disease or infection. If they were not removed they would increase the risk of further infection. This is removed using a fine tube connected to a vacuum to suck the secretions out. It works just like the tube used by dentists to remove saliva. In very ill patients this vacuum tube is in place all the time (page 22).

Pneumothorax

The lungs are like two balloons and pneumothorax is like one balloon popping. This condition is always a risk with people on a ventilator. It can occur when broken ribs tear the lung or as a result of a lung being accidentally punctured or bursting in some way. Instead of the gas going in and out of the lungs it leaks into the chest cavity causing the lungs to collapse and affect the heart. This has to be treated by draining the gases from the cavity with a large tube or sucking it out with a needle and syringe (aspirating) (page 23).

6

Heart disease

The heart is a complex organ that pumps blood around the body and through the lungs. As blood returns from the organs full of waste material and loaded with carbon dioxide it collects in the right atrium of the heart. When that chamber is full it is passed through a one-way valve into the right ventricle. The valve then shuts and the right ventricle pumps blood through another valve and through the lungs.

In the lungs carbon dioxide is taken from the blood and a fresh supply of oxygen collected. The blood then returns to the upper left collecting chamber called the left atrium. From there it passes through a valve to the left ventricle, which in turn pumps it through another valve to the rest of the body through a big blood vessel called the aorta. The cycle then begins again.

There is less work involved in pumping blood through the lungs than in pumping it around the entire body. This means the left side of the heart works harder than the right and generates more pressure. The amount of blood flow through the two portions of the heart is known as the cardiac output and is always the same. It has to be for the heart to work properly.

The differing pressures in the heart are measured in millimetres of mercury (mmHg). This is because the pressure is measured by the height a column of mercury could be

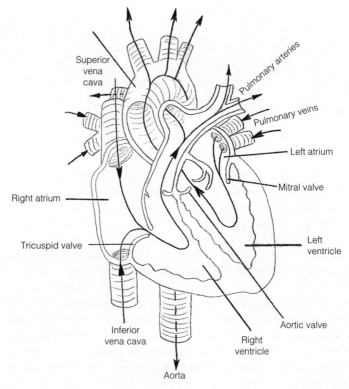

Superior
vena
cava

Pulmonary arteries

Pulmonary veins

Left atrium

Mitral valve

Right atrium

Tricuspid valve

Left
ventricle

Aortic valve

Inferior
vena
cava

Right
ventricle

Aorta

Some parts of the heart.

pushed up by the blood pressure. This is still the unit of measure used, even in electronic hi-tec recording equipment.

There are two blood pressures usually measured. The first is the systolic blood pressure. It is normally around 120 mmHg. This is the force of the blood being squirted into the body from the left ventricle. The second, diastolic pressure, is normally about 80 mmHg. This is pressure remaining in the blood vessels after the heart has stopped its pumping action and the valve out of the left ventricle has shut between heartbeats. These blood pressures are measured with a cuff on the arm or from a tube placed in a small artery at the wrist, groin, or foot.

There is also a different pair of pressures on the right side of the heart which are much lower than the left side. The systolic pressure is normally 20 mmHg and the diastolic pressure 5 mmHg. These can only be measured by placing a tube in the heart – see Swan–Ganz® catheter (Chapter 13, Equipment).

The heart is nearly all muscle and consumes a lot of oxygen itself. It has its own in-built pacemaker known as the sinoatrial node, which is found in the right atrium. This fires off at about 70 beats a minute and stimulates the heart to contract at a coordinated rate. This node reacts to the body's demand for blood and speeds up, or slows down, the heart rate as necessary.

The communication network for the message from the node can be interrupted by disease processes, or can go wrong by itself, and make the heart go faster or slower. Occasionally there may be other areas in the heart that are irritated by disease that then fire off and cause a contraction of the heart. This may or may not be a coordinated contraction. Because this false signal is caused by electrical activity it can be recorded electrically.

One method of recording the heart's activity is the bedside monitor (Chapter 13, Equipment) which just shows basic activity. For a more accurate diagnosis of what is going on in the heart, a 12-lead electrocardiogram (ECG) is often used. The leads are attached at different sites around the body, as the diagram (on page 28) shows, and record and diagnose exactly what and where the heart irregularity is sited.

The most common heart problems that bring patients into an intensive care unit are as follows.

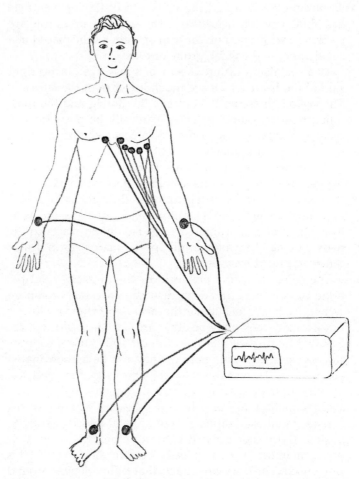

Electrocardiogram. Where the leads from the machine are placed on the body to help find out what is wrong with the heart.

Heart attack

This occurs when the blood supply to the muscle of the heart is cut off. In the western world it is most commonly caused by a hardening of the arteries, and fatty deposits in the arteries, causing them to become blocked. Smoking and diet may play a part in causing it. The patient may complain of a severe pain in the centre of the chest which may also be felt in the arms and neck. The damage to the heart will be diagnosed by the ECG and by measuring the enzymes released into the blood by the damaged heart cells.

When the patient is admitted to an intensive care, or coronary care unit, they can be given a substance to dissolve the blockage and reduce the subsequent damage to the heart. This process is known as thrombolysis. It is not always possible to give this substance to some patients – people who suffer peptic ulcers, or have recently undergone surgery – would not be allowed to have this substance because it would dissolve all the clots, and they might bleed.

, Another priority for staff in the intensive care unit is to deal with any irregularity of the heart caused by the damage. If the heart is going too fast electric shock treatment may be used to stun the heart briefly to allow the heart's own natural pacemaker, the sinoatrial node, to take over. Drugs may also be given to slow it down. If the heart is beating too slowly then drugs may be given to speed it up, or a pacemaker may be necessary.

Cardiac arrest

Cardiac arrest is the phrase used when the heart stops. It can be caused by many things. Heart attack, lack of oxygen, electric shock, drowning, or hypothermia are more usual causes. The aim of ICU staff is to restart the heart as soon as possible, certainly within four minutes. The organ most sensitive to any lack of blood supply is the brain and after four minutes the brain starts to be damaged. The longer the blood supply is stopped the worse this damage may be. Other organs may also be damaged. If the patient has been very cold (for example, if they were suffering from hypothermia, or almost drowned in extremely cold water) their organs can sometimes be undamaged even if their heart has been stopped for much longer.

Intensive care unit staff follow a simple ABC formula for treating the patient. A is for airway, making sure that there is no obstruction to the air passages. B is for breathing, to restore breathing, if necessary by blowing gas into the lungs. C is for circulation, to restart the heart and get the blood circulating.

Circulation may be restored by heart massage. This is done by pressing the breastbone (the sternum) so that the heart is squeezed between the sternum and the spine forcing blood out and around the body. The pressure is then released and the heart fills with blood and the massage is begun again. In order to keep the circulation going like this the heart has to be squeezed about 80 times a minute. Valves in the heart make sure the blood goes in the right direction. Once circulation is supported in this way it is possible to give drugs and electric shocks to restart the heart.

In some patients this will be successful. Those who recover consciousness will then stay in the ICU for a period of observation. Only a few patients remain unconscious. Some of these patients will be admitted to the intensive care unit and placed on a ventilator. Those having difficulty breathing with the ventilator will be kept quiet, still, and sedated for one or two days to give them the best chance of recovery. About half of these will recover and walk out of hospital. The rest will die.

For some patients, those for instance with terminal cancer, resuscitation may not be appropriate as it can just prolong their suffering, and doctors may discuss issuing a 'Do not resuscitate' order. This means that they may feel it is inappropriate to prolong the process of dying. This will usually be discussed with the patient, their relatives, or both in advance. It can allow the patient and their family to say goodbye properly and is often chosen instead of a long drawn-out and often more unpleasant period before dying.

Viral disease

Minute organisms may attack the muscle of the heart weakening it. This is very difficult to treat and may need a transplant.

Direct injury

This is usually as a result of a road traffic accident, stabbing, or gun-shot injury. Surgery may be needed to repair the heart, followed by a period of care in an intensive care unit.

Heart failure

This is not the same as cardiac arrest. This happens when the heart is not working properly. Either the left or right ventricle can fail, or both can fail together. This can be caused by any of the diseases mentioned before.

Failure of the right ventricle can be caused by lung disease. This makes the right ventricle work harder than it is designed to do and sometimes it fails under the strain of the heavy workload. Then blood does not go to the left side of the heart. Pressure builds up in the blood vessels leading to the right side of the heart. Fluid then tends to leak out of the veins and into the surrounding tissues. The tissues can become boggy. This is called oedema. This is often noticed first with patients' ankles swelling.

When the left side of the heart fails pressure builds up in the blood vessels leading to it. These blood vessels are in the lungs. Fluid leaks from them into the lungs. They become boggy (pulmonary oedema). The lungs become stiff and breathing becomes difficult.

7

Kidney failure

Kidney failure (renal failure) in patients on an intensive care unit is normally sudden and associated with major illness or injury. There are many causes of kidney failure. The most common causes are:

- shock – after infection or severe blood loss from injury or surgery
- as part of a multiorgan failure – explained more fully in Chapter 12.
- Some forms of poisoning and drugs
- diseases of the immune system
- diseases affecting the blood vessels that lead to the kidneys
- an obstruction to the outflow from the kidneys

Kidney failure in a critically ill patient can usually be successfully treated. If the patient recovers, but the kidneys are still not working properly, then long-term dialysis or transplantation may be considered.

The two kidneys are located either side of the spine in the lower back. They are responsible for maintaining the right quantities of water and essential salts in the body. They also excrete from the body, in urine, various poisons including drugs and their by-products.

Kidneys are very efficient filters. They can process 180 litres of water, salts, and poisons each day. Most of the

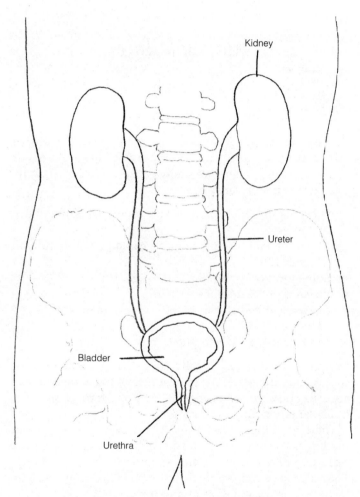

Where the kidneys are found in the body.

filtered water and some of the salts are reabsorbed into the body. The filter in the kidney is called the glomerulus. The filtered liquid is passed through tubes called tubules. They are responsible for sorting the salts to be retained and passing out the poisons. After this the fluid goes into the collecting ducts which join together. These eventually form a single tube, the ureter, which takes the excess liquid and waste away from the kidney to the bladder. The bladder is merely a store for the waste fluid which is passed out of the body as urine. Kidney function is regulated by both its own control mechanisms and the brain.

Most intensive care patients who are very seriously ill or unconscious will have a tube called a catheter draining urine from the bladder. The catheter goes from the bladder, along the urethra, to the normal urinary opening and then into a collecting bag.

When the kidneys 'fail' one of three things can happen.

- Virtually no urine is passed. This is anuric renal failure.
- Too much urine is passed because the tubules malfunction and liquid is not reabsorbed properly. This is polyuric failure.
- Urine of poor quality is made, in normal quantities. Poisons are not filtered out.

In an intensive care unit one of the kidneys' functions is routinely tested every day by measuring the fluids passing into the patient against the amount passing out. This is all part of an essential daily check on the fluid balance of all intensive care patients. This is because the amount of fluid lost from the body includes urine (if any), sweat, stomach drains, and diarrhoea – in fact any fluid leaving the body. It is not easy accurately to measure the fluids passing out of a body each day, so in many ICUs patients are regularly weighed as well. There are regular daily blood checks to test the levels of essential salts such as sodium, potassium, and urea, which is a by-product of protein and creatinine – in turn a by-product of muscles.

The sodium and potassium tests will show how well the kidneys are working. Increasing levels of urea and creatinine usually indicate kidney failure. Another sign of kidney failure is a general swelling of the patient's skin (oedema). This indicates too much fluid is being retained and not passed through the kidneys. To establish how bad kidney failure may be, tests are carried out on the urine – if there is any – to discover the levels of sodium and creatinine and the concentration of the urine.

The methods of treatment depend upon the severity and type of kidney failure. If no urine is being passed then the patient will need kidney support in the form of haemodialysis or haemofiltration, or a combination of both. Both systems work by purifying the blood. (This is more fully described in Chapter 13, Equipment).

If urine is still being made, either in excessive or normal quantities, treatment is slightly easier. Doctors have a variety of manoeuvres in these cases to try and avoid dialysis, including:

- Restrict the amount of fluid going in, then balance that amount with the quantity coming out.
- Restrict the amount of protein-containing food given to the patient. Protein in food is an important cause of urea in blood and one of the poisons excreted by the kidney (but see Chapter 16 for the dangerous effects of starvation).
- Restrict the amount of potassium going into the patient by altering their diet. For example, grapes, oranges, and chocolate contain enormous amounts of potassium and these will be cut from the diet of someone with kidney failure.

An overdose of potassium can be fatal. It will stop the heart. Patients with renal failure will receive little or no potassium in their diet or feeds. Difficulty can arise, however, because potassium is a by-product of muscle and other tissues wasting. This can happen as a result of a severe injury or infection. This production of potassium is dangerous. Dialysis will be used to reduce this level of potassium.

Doctors treating patients with kidney failure take great care with the drugs they prescribe. This is because drugs can become poisonous, or can produce poisonous substances, which the affected kidneys are unable to remove or filter properly.

8

Liver and gut disease

The liver and gut work together. When you eat food it is held initially in the stomach where acids attack it, purify it, and partly break it down. The food then passes to the small bowel, which is about 6–7 metres (20 feet) long and 4 centimetres ($1\frac{1}{2}$ inches) wide. In the small bowel it is broken down further by enzymes secreted from the pancreas. This food is then absorbed by the small bowel and passed along a system of veins to the liver. After the liver has done its work the blood containing its processed food is passed to the body by another system of veins. This type of venous system is called a portal system. When the absorbed food arrives through the veins at the liver, the liver then turns the food into energy needed by the rest of the body.

The food that has not been absorbed from the small bowel and passed to the liver passes on through the gut into the section of intestine known as the large bowel. This is about a metre (3–4 feet) long and about 6–7 centimetres ($2\frac{1}{2}$ inches) in diameter. In this section most of the moisture is absorbed, leaving fibre and other waste material. The large bowel stores the remaining matter as faeces ready to be excreted.

Liver disease

The liver is one of the most complex organs in the body and has an amazing 1500 separate functions. That's why

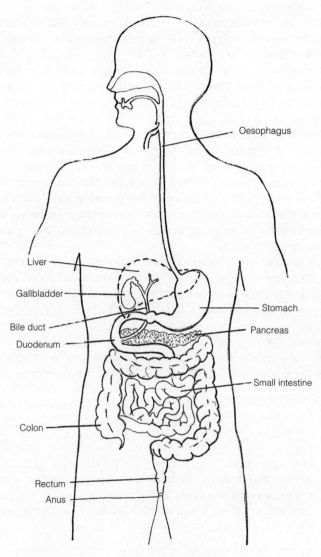

The digestive system.

it's impossible, even with today's advanced technology, to create an artificial liver. It is possible to transplant a liver, but because the organ is so complex it sometimes doesn't work well in its new body.

Patients may be admitted to an intensive care unit because of liver disease. This can be caused by a viral infection, a bacterial infection, alcohol abuse, or exposure to poisons such as drug overdoses. For many diseases the cause is still unknown. Liver disease is characterized by a jaundiced appearance in the patient. Their skin and the whites of their eyes turn yellow. It can also be accompanied by abnormal blood clotting or internal bleeding, particularly if there is an obstruction to the portal blood flow. The obstruction can cause a pressure build-up in those veins which can burst around the gullet (oesophagus) and cause a major haemorrhage.

A patient with internal bleeding may vomit blood (haematemesis). They may also become unconscious. This is called hepatic encephalopathy. Liver failure can also lead to low blood sugar levels that can lead to brain damage and death.

Liver disease will affect almost every other organ in the body, especially the heart, lungs, and kidneys. As a result of liver disease people can suffer a whole range of conditions such as:

- lack of blood clotting agents (clotting factors).
- coma (encephalopathy)
- hepato-renal syndrome, when the kidneys fail because of liver disease
- hepato-pulmonary syndrome, when a disease of the liver can cause the lungs to fail
- cardiomyopathy, when disease of the liver can cause the muscles of the heart to fail

In an intensive care unit when liver failure occurs, or a patient is admitted with liver failure, they will be observed to see how they progress. If they start to fall unconscious (encephalopathy) they may need to be put on a ventilator.

Any bleeding will be stopped if possible by giving artificial clotting agents such as special plasma (FFP). If there is internal bleeding the doctor will look inside the body with a fibreoptic instrument (an endoscope) and inject a clotting agent directly into the veins that are bleeding. If blood breaks down in the body it can cause poisons to be released into the body which affect the brain. Blood is cleared out of the gut by giving laxatives.

Doctors and nurses in the intensive care unit measure blood glucose and give top-up vitamins to assist a person suffering from liver failure. In a few serious cases a liver transplant may be considered.

Gut disease

Other organs in the food-processing chain can be affected by disease. For example there are many diseases which affect the stomach. The most common ailment in intensive care patients is ulcers which rapidly form on the stomach wall. They are usually caused by stress, just as they are in someone with a high-powered job. Stress can also cause ulcers in the duodenum which is situated at the start of the small bowel.

Stress can also be caused by burns or kidney failure, or the strain of being on a ventilator. Ulcers can be treated with some drugs. Fortunately, the occurrence of ulcers has decreased in recent years because of the drug treatment given to patients in intensive care and improved resuscitation techniques.

Diarrhoea is a very serious problem in the severely ill. It can be caused by the disease that brought the patient to the intensive care unit or an infection, most commonly *Clostridium difficile*, a bacteria. Another cause of diarrhoea can be irritation caused by the tube feed (Chapter 16, Feeding).

Antibiotics given to treat an infection can also cause diarrhoea. This happens when the antibiotics interfere with the bacteria which are normally present in the intestines and help with the breakdown of food passing through.

Doctors and nurses will try and stop the diarrhoea because it is most uncomfortable and embarrassing for the patient and is potentially dangerous. A patient with diarrhoea loses fluids, essential salts, and food, and can develop sores around the backside (anal excoriation).

The pancreas sends out powerful enzymes into the gut to break down the food and enable it to be absorbed and passed to the liver. If the pancreas fails because of viral disease, gall stones, or some injury, then these powerful enzymes may be released into the abdominal cavity rather than the gut. They can cause an immense amount of damage as they start breaking down the body itself. Pancreatitis is a very serious disease and must be treated immediately.

The other function of the pancreas is to secrete insulin into the blood. This is the hormone which controls the glucose concentration in the blood. Anything that inhibits this function can cause diabetes. From time to time patients will be admitted into the intensive care unit because of diabetic emergencies.

9

Accidents

The most common types of injuries from accidents that put patients in intensive care are those to the head and chest.

Head injuries

Patients with serious head injuries from an accident are often treated in intensive care units.

The brain swells after injury, just as a thumb will swell if hit by a hammer. The swelling can be made worse if the patient coughs, strains, or has their airway obstructed in any way. The act of straining or coughing drives blood to the brain, increasing the pressure and the swelling. Because the brain is enclosed inside the skull (a bony box) this limits the area in which the brain can be allowed to swell. If it swells too much it will cut off its own blood supply damaging the brain. That is why it is important to stop the swelling.

The aim of treatment in the intensive care unit is to reduce or prevent the brain swelling. This is done by the following methods.

- Stop the coughing by making sure the airway is clear at all times, by placing a tracheal tube in the trachea under anaesthetic and temporarily paralysing the patient with a muscle relaxant.

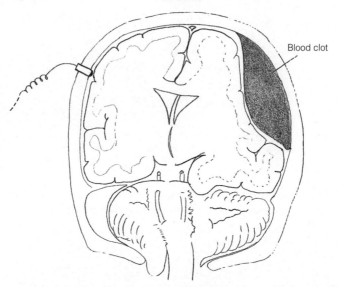
Blood clot

The brain being compressed by swelling and a blood clot. A pressure-measuring 'bolt' is also shown.

- Lessen the amount of swelling by giving dehydrating agents such as mannitol which causes excess urine to be passed (Chapter 15, Drugs).
- Insert a device for measuring the pressure in the brain. This is called a 'bolt'.
- Give other drugs to reduce brain pressure, such as thiopentone. This drug, and others like it, may also reduce oxygen requirements of the cells.

Where a muscle relaxant has been given it will also be necessary to place the patient on a ventilator.

A lot of head injuries are diagnosed with a CT scanner — a computerized tomography scanner (Chapter 13, Equipment). Repeated scans may be necessary to see what has happened inside the brain. This sort of treatment will go on for one to seven days and in some instances longer, depending on the individual practice of the intensive care unit. The treatment may be periodically interrupted so that the patient can be woken up for state of their brain to be assessed.

Sometimes as a result of a head injury a blood clot may form in the brain. This may need to be removed by an operation.

The treatment of brain injury may affect the way other injuries are treated. Unfortunately, patients with injuries to the brain often require prolonged rehabilitation and support long after they have recovered from their other injuries.

Chest injuries

For the lungs to work properly they need their cage of 12 ribs intact. The movement of the ribs during the act of breathing creates a vacuum in the chest that sucks air into the lungs through the airways. Damage to several ribs can seriously affect this mechanical action making breathing and coughing difficult and painful. Most accident victims with chest injuries that include broken ribs need effective pain relief by means of a continuous epidural (page 75). A few may need a breathing machine to help them. The lungs can also be bruised in an accident. This causes swelling which interferes with the passage of oxygen into the blood in the lungs. The swelling is reduced by giving diuretics (page 80).

The heart and major blood vessels can be damaged by chest injuries. These will need urgent surgery and intensive care.

Abdominal injuries

Serious injuries to the lower trunk can be life threatening because of bleeding from abdominal organs such as the spleen and liver. Damage to other organs, such as the stomach and intestines, may spill their contents and cause peritonitis or abscesses. This may need an operation and intensive care afterwards.

10

Neurological diseases

The brain and the spinal cord are known as the central nervous system. It can be affected by many diseases. The most common causes are brain injury, something going drastically wrong with the body's chemistry or major organs, poisoning, or some infections, such as meningitis. While the cause is being diagnosed, general bodily functions such as the breathing and circulation are supported.

A patient can arrive in an intensive care unit having continual, uncontrollable fits, despite attempts to treat them, or they can develop in the intensive unit. This again is a sign of something seriously wrong with the central nervous system. Fits can occur with epilepsy and meningitis, after injury, or when something goes wrong with the body's chemistry, and after a stroke or brain haemorrhage. They can be difficult to treat.

The treatment of the fits is to stop them. Usually the patient has to be put to sleep with drugs like phenytoin, diazepam, or thiopentone. It may also be necessary to temporarily paralyse the patient to stop muscular twitching. A combination of these two treatments means that the patient will have to be put on a ventilator, as they will not be able to breathe unaided.

Guillain–Barré syndrome

This is a disease that does not affect the central nervous system but the rest of the nerves that control the muscles. It usually follows a minor viral infection but it is not known what causes it. Victims complain of a tingling sensation in their fingers and toes which rapidly progresses to a weakness that eventually affects the muscles used for breathing. In some patients this is so serious they will need to be put on to a ventilator until they recover from the disease. This may take weeks.

Most patients get better with time. Sometimes the blood may have some of the agents that cause the syndrome taken out of it by a process called plasmapheresis. This means literally taking all the plasma out of the blood system and putting new plasma in.

There is a national support group for patients and families of patients with Guillain–Barré syndrome and the staff of the intensive care unit will be happy to tell you how to get in touch with the group.

Myasthenia gravis

This is a disease that can cause severe weakness in the 'voluntary' muscles – those muscles you tell to move – and particularly the eyes, throat, and chest.

The disease causes the body's own immune system to attack some of the 'receptors' in the muscles which receive instructions from the brain through nerves. This disrupts the signals to the muscles which tell them to work.

Sufferers can look as if they are 'half-asleep' as the eyelids refuse to open fully. Sufferers complain of losing strength, double vision, and difficulty in swallowing. As the disease progresses difficulties with breathing can develop.

What sets off this disease is unknown but it can be made worse by a chest infection. Sometimes anaesthetics and other drugs can aggravate the condition and the sufferer has to be admitted to an intensive care unit. There the patient's breathing will be aided, if necessary, and drugs adjusted to help the muscles function better.

In some severe attacks doctors will try and filter off the proteins in the blood that cause problems with the receptors in the muscles.

11

Poisoning

Patients are frequently admitted to intensive care units as a result of poisoning. This can happen in various ways. They can be poisoned as a result of an industrial accident or an accident in the home involving the swallowing of some toxic substance. Some patients may have poisoned themselves in an attempt to commit suicide.

Poison victims often have shallow and difficult breathing. Their heart may be poisoned and may not pump very well and have an irregular rhythm. The patient's temperature can also be abnormal, either very hot or very cold. The poisoned patient can also be dehydrated because they may have been lying unconscious for a long time or passed a lot of urine. The general body chemistry can also be affected. Liver failure can also result. Tests are done on the blood and urine to measure the concentration of drugs or find out what drugs may have been taken if the poison is not known.

The priority is to establish a clear airway and remove any poisons in the stomach if they have been taken by mouth.

Staff give drugs that may combat, reduce or even reverse some of the effects of the poison. These are called antagonists. For example in the case of paracetamol poisoning it is possible to administer the drug N-acetyl cysteine. This lessens poisonous by-products of paracetamol being made in the body, making instead a harmless by-product which will be safely passed from the poison victim, if given early enough.

Some drugs can be removed from the body by kidney dialysis and other similar techniques.

12

Multi-organ failure

Some patients in intensive care, who were originally admitted suffering the failure of one vital organ, can suffer multi-organ failure.

The shut-down of one vital organ can bring on a domino effect that causes other vital organs to fail. Patients can suffer the devastating effect of having any combination of their vital organs failing. The usual combination seen in patients in the intensive care unit is lungs, heart, kidney, liver, and gut all failing at the same time.

The most common cause of multi-organ failure is a severe life-threatening infection, although any major injury, illness, or poisoning can cause it. Infection or any of the other causes of multi-organ failure can release throughout the body 'inflammatory mediators'. These normally carry messages between cells on how they should react when attacked by disease, injury, or infection. But in some cases of severe life-threatening infection excess quantities of these messengers are released. The spread of the excess inflammatory mediators by the blood to all parts of the body causes cells to stop working properly, including those in vital organs. Shock (see Chapter 4) can also cause the release of those inflammatory mediators.

One of the greatest problems with multi-organ failure is that the devastating effects do not appear for two or three days after the release of inflammatory mediators. By then it is very difficult to treat and has a high mortality rate – a large number of people will not survive it.

The only treatment for multi-organ failure is to support those organs that have failed and to remove any source of sepsis. Keeping multi-organ failure patients alive is more complicated than flying a jumbo jet and there is no auto-pilot or computer assistance. The treatment includes vigor-ous resuscitation by ensuring that there is enough blood in the circulatory system, enough oxygen in that blood, and the heart is pumping well. At the same time doctors have to ensure that the right antibiotics are being given and any surgery necessary to mend broken bones, or remove the source of infection, is carried out.

Small intensive care units, which have a patient suffer-ing multi-organ failure will have to transfer those patients to a larger unit where there are experienced staff and the equipment to cope with the extremely complicated support of all the bodily functions.

There is a vast amount of research currently being conducted to try and find drugs to stop the excess of inflammatory mediators being released or to try and reduce their devastating effect on the vital organs. Studies are also underway to discover a means of removing the dangerous mediators from the blood.

ARDS (Acute respiratory distress syndrome)

ARDS is commonly a part of multi-organ failure and is also seen in patients with a lung injury or severe infection or injury to other parts of the body. Both lungs become stiff, hard, and fibrous and are difficult to inflate. The patient usually has to be supported by a ventilator as the lungs do not absorb oxygen properly. ARDS is also thought to be caused by the release of excess inflammatory mediators. Unfortunately many patients die from ARDS. Trials have started of experimental treatments for ARDS including the use of a machine to bypass the lungs and put oxygen into the blood outside of the body. Other trials using an extremely low concentration of nitric oxide gas in the breathing mixture have shown temporary benefits.

13

Equipment

Ventilator

The ventilator simply takes oxygen and other gas or air from a supply, blends them in a required quantity, and passes the mixture on to the patient. The normal amount of oxygen in the air we breath is 21%. The ventilator can administer up to 100% oxygen, depending on how sick the patient's lungs may be. The ventilator transfers the mix to the patient through a tube inserted in the trachea. A filter on the tube traps bacteria and warms and moistens the oxygen and gas as necessary.

The ventilator contains a pump, a gas store, and various electronic controls. Together these enable the oxygen mix to be passed to the patient in the required amount and at the required pressure in a breathing pattern set by medical staff. The ventilator also has a PEEP valve (see p. 20) which controls the pressure inside the lungs and makes sure it never reaches zero. This prevents the lungs collapsing or sticking together. (See IPPV, SIMV, PEEP, CPAP, and ASB in Chapter 5, Breathing difficulties.)

Digital displays on the ventilator show:

- the amount of oxygen in the lungs
- the amount of oxygen in the mix reaching the lungs
- the pressure of gases in the lungs
- the number of breaths being taken per minute.

54

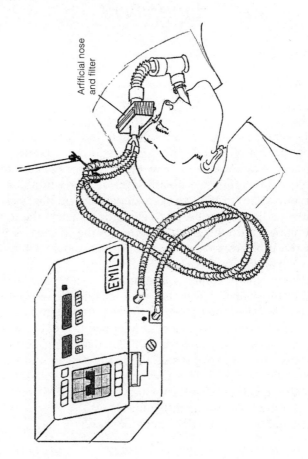

Artificial nose
and filter

The ventilator (breathing machine).
Also shown is the connecting tubing and the artificial nose and filter.

These machines are very expensive and cost between £15 000 and £20 000 each.

In some intensive care units the ventilator and other key pieces of equipment may well be labelled with a name such as; Daisy, Tony, or Mary. They are named so that the various parts of each piece of equipment are easily identified after cleaning or repair. Names are also easier to remember than serial numbers and help personalize an area packed with hi-tec electrical equipment.

Breathing support can also be given through a 'pilot's' type of mask (see CPAP in Chapter 5, Breathing difficulties).

Monitors

Modern monitors can keep an electronic watch on up to 20 different bodily and organ functions and display them on a screen. They are also equipped with visual and audible alarms should anything start to go wrong with those functions.

Electrical activity in the heart is displayed using an electrocardiogram. Electrical activity is detected from three sensors attached to the chest. The heartbeat and blood pressure can be monitored from a tube inserted into an artery in the wrist, foot, elbow, or groin. The tube goes to an electronic gadget called a transducer that changes the blood pressure into an electronic signal that can be displayed. This tube will also be fitted with a small tap so blood samples can be easily taken for analysis. It is also possible to measure blood pressure without using tubes and needles. The usual 'wrap-around' and 'pump-up' pressure machine used by doctors can be strapped to the patient's arm and linked to an electronic monitor.

A tube inserted into the body and sited just above the top right chamber of the heart, the right atrium, and linked to a

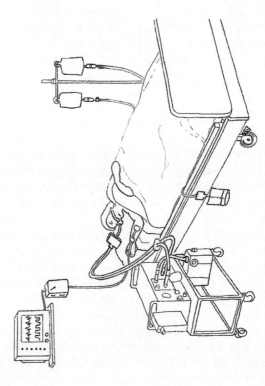

Monitors around a patient. The screen above the patient shows an electrocardiogram and blood pressures measured from an artery in the wrist and around the heart. Also shown is a device for collecting and measuring the urine (hanging from the bed), a ventilator and two bags of intravenous fluid.

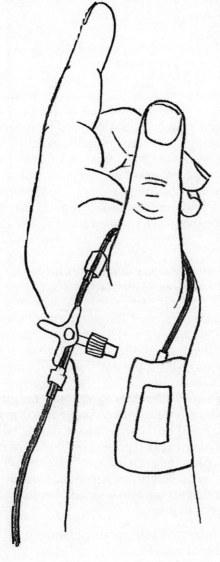

Arterial line. A small tube inserted into an artery in the wrist, elbow, groin, or foot. It is used to measure blood pressure and take blood for analysis.

monitor displays central venous pressure or right atrial pressure (see p. 56).

Pulse oximeter

This is a clever gadget that can be attached to the ears, nose, fingers, or toes. It shines three small beams of red light through the blood vessels. It then displays on a screen the heart rate and the amount of oxygen in the blood. The lights measure the redness of the blood from beat to beat and that tells the machine the amount of oxygen being carried in the blood. This machine can also give out an audible tone that changes with the level of oxygen being recorded. The normal oxygen saturation (SpO_2) is a value greater than 85% (p. 59).

Pulmonary artery flotation catheter or Swan–Ganz® catheter

This is a tube that is inserted through a neck vein or the femoral vein in the groin. A small balloon is inflated at its tip. It is then floated through the veins to the heart where it passes through the right atrium and the right ventricle and on into the pulmonary artery.

Once in place a cold solution is injected into the tube and it then passes through the heart and past a fine thermometer sited near the end of the tube. Blood mixing with the cold solution is cooled very slightly. This slight decrease in temperature is passed to a computer which then calculates how many litres of blood are being pumped from the heart per minute. This device can also be used to measure many other things. For example:

- the amount of oxygen being absorbed into the body
- the state of blood vessels

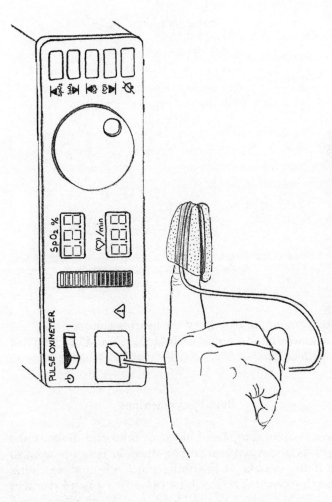

Pulse oximeter: this measures the amount of oxygen in the blood from a small sensor on the finger or elsewhere.

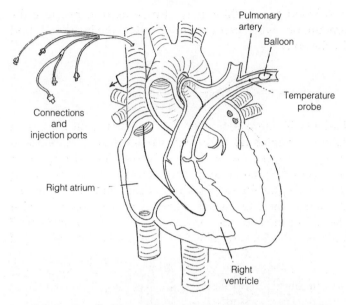

A Swan–Ganz® catheter. This tube passes through the heart and measures many of its functions.

- the amount of blood that the heart is pumping
- a guide to the amount of fluid that should be given to a patient.

Blood gas machines

These analyse samples of blood or fluid and measure the amounts of oxygen and carbon dioxide. They are used to see if the patient is breathing efficiently and receiving enough oxygen. The machine can also measure the acid and alkaline levels in the blood, which can show if the patient has suffered metabolic problems.

A blood gas machine may also be used to measure the amount of oxygen being pumped out by the heart and used by the body.

Gastric tonometry

Patients in intensive care can die from multiple organ failure (Chapter 12, Multi-organ failure). As a response to being seriously ill the body diverts blood from lesser organs to the vital organs – the heart, lungs, and brain – as the body fights for survival. If this goes on for too long the barriers in the intestines that keep dangerous bacteria from the rest of the body can break down. These harmful bacteria then pass into the blood and can cause infections that can attack the vital organs.

As the blood supply to the intestines reduces the level of acid in these organs increases. By checking these acid levels with a gastric tonometer the medical staff can take action with drugs to maintain the barriers in the intestines. The amount of acid in the stomach is measured by putting a tube into the stomach with a small balloon on the end filled with a salt solution. The level of acid in the salt solution measured by a blood gas machine, coupled with a blood sample, can tell medical staff the state of those vital barriers and what action to take to maintain them.

Syringe pumps

Potent drugs are diluted and put in a large syringe which is clamped into a syringe pump. The electronic pump then gradually pushes the drug through a tube and through a plastic tube in a vein. The amount the patient receives each hour is prescribed by medical staff and set on the machine. Alarms, both visual and audible, will sound if anything

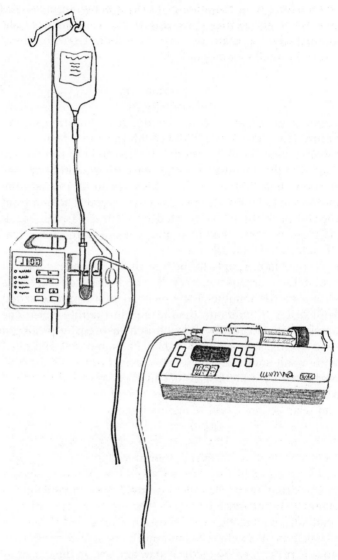

Infusion and syringe pumps. Used to give drugs and fluids accurately.

goes wrong with the amount of drug being administered and when the syringe has almost run out of drug. The pumps allow accurate delivery of concentrated solutions of drugs in small volumes of fluid.

Infusion pump

This is used for larger volumes of drugs, or for other fluids such as blood, saline, or feed. Some infusion pumps can operate two separate 'drips' at once while measuring the amount in millilitres per hour passing to the patient. Any number of pumps can be used as required on a single patient. They are all fitted with alarms (p. 62).

Dialysis machines

A kidney dialysis machine, usually found in an intensive care unit, pumps blood in a tube from the patient via a vein in the chest, neck, or groin. The blood is then passed through an artificial kidney which removes the waste and poisons. The blood is then rewarmed to body temperature and passed back along a tube to the patient. This process is called continuous veno-venous haemodiafiltration.

Blood can also be taken from an artery using the patient's own heart to pump the blood through the filter and is then restored to a vein. This process is called continuous arterio-venous haemodiafiltration.

These types of dialysis both differ from the system in renal units where the treatment lasts for a few hours and is given usually every other day.

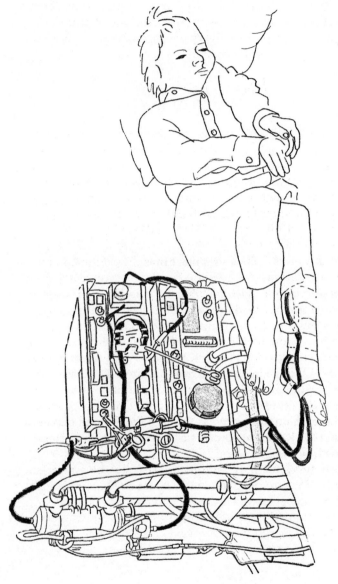

The most commonest form of renal dialysis equipment used in intensive care units, continuous veno-venous haemodiafiltration (CVVHD).

14

Investigations

All day, every day, routine investigations are carried out on patients in intensive care units. These tests are in addition to the frequent visits to the bedside by doctors and constant monitoring by nurses and machines.

Many of these investigations involve the analysis of various samples of blood and urine and the examination of the chest and other parts of the body by X-rays. They are designed to enable staff to know what is going on inside the patient in addition to the vast array of hi-tec equipment surrounding the patient.

Tests will show how treatment of the patient's injury or disease is progressing. They will enable doctors and nurses to make subtle changes to the drugs, food and drink, or liquids being given to the patient, and enable them to maintain the correct course of treatment and the chemical and fluid balance in the body. They will also enable medical staff to decide on any further courses of treatment necessary, such as dialysis.

Occasionally there is some unexplained problem, or a source of disease or infection that has not been located, and one of a number of special investigations may have to be carried out in addition to the daily routine investigations.

Briefly, the most common routine investigations carried out in an intensive care unit are as follows.

Blood tests

Some blood tests measure several functions.

- *Blood gases* The levels of carbon dioxide and oxygen in the blood will tell medical staff how well the lungs are working and how much oxygen may be needed by a patient.

The normal amount of oxygen in the arterial blood (PaO_2) is greater than 8 kPa or 60 mmHg. Similarly, the amount of carbon dioxide in the arterial blood ($PaCO_2$) is about 4.5 kPa or 33 mmHg. The two units of measurement (mmHg or kPa) measure the same thing but are different in size – it's like measuring distance in miles or kilometres.

- *Acid or alkaline levels* These levels in the blood will indicate the state of the kidneys and other organs. The various levels also tell doctors how well an injury or disease is responding to treatment.

- *Potassium* It is essential to measure the levels of potassium in the blood. Too little will cause the heart to beat irregularly. Too much can cause the heart to stop.

- *Blood glucose* This test is carried out frequently as levels can change rapidly. High levels of blood glucose can be created as a reaction to injury or trauma or drugs.

Sometimes a high level is caused by too much feeding. If it is too high some insulin may be given. If it is too low then insulin may be stopped or glucose given.

- *Poisons* Levels of naturally occurring poisons, such as urea and creatinine, are measured regularly. The amount of these substances in the blood will show how well the kidneys are functioning.

- *Salts (electrolytes)* The level of these, in particular sodium, will depend upon the amounts of water and plasma given to a patient. The concentration of sodium will indicate whether a patient is becoming dehydrated or not.

- *Clotting* There are at least 13 different factors required to occur in a chain reaction to start blood clotting. By testing some of those factors, and the substances involved, doctors can spot what may be going wrong with the blood clotting, where it's going wrong and why. They will usually examine the levels of prothrombin, fibrinogen, and the numbers of platelets.

- *Enzymes* Organs that are damaged all release different enzymes. Measuring these will indicate which organs are damaged and how badly. For example, in heart attacks creatinine kinease is measured.

- *Liver function* Natural proteins in the blood are produced by the liver and changes will show how different parts of this vital and complex organ are working. Measuring the proteins prothrombin and albumin shows how well the liver is working. Measuring the level of bilirubin in the blood shows how efficiently the liver is excreting material.

Enzymes, such as alkaline phosphatase and ALT (alanine aminotransferase), are found in the blood when the liver is damaged. The amount of these enzymes indicates how bad the damage is in certain circumstances.

- *White blood cells* A count of the white blood cells that fight infection will show how much infection there is, how well it is being dealt with, whether drugs or antibiotics may be required, and whether they are working.

- *Bone marrow function* The platelet count will also show how efficiently the bone marrow is working in producing new platelets.

- *Weight checks* A sudden weight loss or gain would indicate a change in the water balance of a patient.

- *Food required* Tests of the blood levels of glucose and albumin, coupled with the patient's weight, will give doctors and nurses an idea of how much to feed a patient.

Urine

Samples of urine are frequently tested to see how well the kidneys are functioning. Urine can also be analysed in a similar way to blood to show levels of various chemicals and proteins. This will indicate how well treatment is progressing.

- *Urine concentration* This will show the water balance of the body and enable the fluid levels to be controlled as necessary.

- *Protein concentration* Concentrations of different proteins can show how various diseases are progressing.

- *Blood in the urine* Detecting blood in the urine can indicate something that may be wrong with a kidney.

- *Acid and alkaline levels* These can help establish the levels of essential salts and electrolytes in a patient's body, particularly potassium.

X-rays

Chest X-rays are often taken every day. They will show if the lungs are damaged and indicate any diseases affecting them. The X-rays will show any air leaks from the lungs (pneumothorax) that may need to be treated. They will also show the present position of the various tubes inserted into the chest.

Special investigations

There are literally hundreds of special investigations that could be carried out for various reasons. They are not usually carried out unless they are absolutely necessary for the welfare of the patient. The most common of these special investigations are explained below.

- *Electrocardiograph (ECG)* For this investigation six wires are attached to the chest and four on the limbs and a print-out of the heart's electrical activity is obtained. From these doctors can work out how much damage may have been done to the heart and where it's damaged. It will also show if the heart is beating errati-cally (Chapter 6, Heart disease).

- *Echocardiograph* This beams ultrasound waves at the heart rather like the scan a pregnant woman has to examine the unborn baby. This enables the doctors to see the heart at work.

- *Electroencephalogram (EEG)* This involves placing eight or more electrodes on the head. This is usually carried out on an unconscious patient to check the brain's func-tions or to find out why a patient is having fits.

- *CT scan* One of the most widely used pieces of equip-ment for people with head injuries was a CT scanner (computerized tomography scanner). It may some-times be referred to as a CAT scanner, as its old name was a computerized axial tomography scanner. This is a sophisticated X-ray machine linked to a computer and is capable of showing cross sections of the brain and other organs. Abnormalities such as haemorrhages, tumours, or bruising show up as lighter or darker areas of the brain. CT scans of other parts of the body can locate areas of pus or fluid that can be drained with a very fine tube without the need for an operation. Doctors can use the CT scan of the body to find areas of internal bleeding or locate an abscess or tumour. The CT scanner shows up damage from this disease or injury and helps the doctor plan treatment.

A general hospital will often have a CT scanner and it is possible that a patient suffering from a head injury can be given a scan at his local hospital and the picture obtained sent down a telephone line to a specialist neurosurgeon in a major hospital. The surgeon can then study the X-rays and decide if it is necessary for the patient to be transferred to a specialist neuro-intensive care unit.

• *White cell scan* In this investigation a few of the patient's white blood cells are removed and 'tagged' with a harmless dose of a radiatioactive marker. When the cells are put back into the patient they will collect around and locate hidden infection sites. A camera that detects very low levels of radiation is used to see this.

• *Ultrasound scan* Ultrasound scanners are regularly used to look at various internal organs and locate fluid collections. It is particularly useful because the machine is portable and can be brought to the patient. For many other tests the patient needs to be moved to the machine.

- *Surgery* Some special investigations can only be carried out by operating and actually looking at the injured or diseased area.

15

Drugs

Medical science is advancing at an ever-increasing rate, but there is still no one 'quick fix' drug to kill the infection or disease that may afflict the seriously ill patient. A considerable amount of unsuccessful research has been devoted to finding a 'magic bullet' drug that can be aimed at a specific target in the body. Nature can be too clever. Bacteria, for example, can swiftly mutate as they multiply, so their 'offspring' become resistant to the killing properties of antibiotics.

A patient in intensive care may need several drugs to combat infection, other drugs to cope with problems such as pain, anxiety, and heart irregularities, as well as the drugs to treat the initial condition causing them to be fighting for life.

There are additional problems with the use of drugs in the critically ill. These problems can cause the drugs to act at a slower rate, work for a longer period, and take a longer time to work their way out of the body.

Drugs passing through a patient eventually arrive at the liver which changes their chemical structure and stops them working. They are then disposed of through the kidneys. In a critically ill patient the liver may not be working properly so the drugs take longer to be processed into their by-product (metabolite) and passed to the kidneys. The patient may also have suffered shock which slows down the amount of drug-laden blood reaching the liver. Most drugs given to the seriously ill are injected directly to the blood through a fine tube (intravenously). This is because drugs given by mouth may not be absorbed by a damaged or diseased stomach and digestive system, or the digestive system may not be working properly through illness or the effect of the other drugs.

A common way of giving drugs is to inject them into muscle. But drugs are rarely injected this way into seriously ill patients for several reasons – for one thing with the amount of drugs needed they could soon resemble a pin cushion. Drugs which may usually be injected into muscles of normal patients are also not injected into intensive care patients because of their reduced muscle blood flow and poor blood clotting. The low muscle blood flow means they won't be absorbed. An injection could cause bleeding into the muscle (haematoma).

Drugs are not injected under the skin in the seriously ill because the reduced blood flow would not carry the drugs through the body. Drugs are occasionally given by suppository through the back passage (rectum) from where they are absorbed into the body. Giving drugs intravenously is the fastest and most reliable delivery method.

Some drugs are given by bolus dose. This means that the amount needed is measured in a syringe and slowly squirted into the tube over a period of between 30 seconds and five minutes, depending upon the type of drug. Other drugs, often those that work for a shorter time, have to be given by a continuous slow process. They can reach the body from a drip bag suspended over the bed and controlled by a pump, or they can arrive via a concentrated solution controlled by a syringe pump (Chapter 13, Equipment). Some drugs will need to be fed continuously to the patient, such as adrenaline, to keep up blood pressure. Other drugs are given in short bursts.

The tube bringing the drugs to the patient may be inserted into a vein in the hand, arm, or foot (peripherally). These should usually carry only those drugs that do not irritate the lining of the vein. A problem can arise if the tube wears away the thin vein wall. This can be difficult to detect. The drug can then damage skin and tissue which could die and cause a serious wound. To avoid this, with drugs that can be very irritating, the tube can be inserted into a larger vein in the chest or groin. Here the blood flows faster and dilutes the drug more making it less of an irritant. Some of the drugs being administered this way are very concentrated and therefore very irritant. If the drugs had to be diluted before being administered, enormous quantities of liquid would be needed.

Painkilling drugs can be controlled by the patient in some circumstances. The patient can simply use a button connected to a "pain pump" to give themselves a dose as and when they feel the need. There are controls to stop an overdose. Pain killing drugs may also be given as epidural injections (into the spine) like those often received by pregnant women in labour.

We will now give a brief outline of the types of drug used in intensive care. Some drugs have more than one effect and will appear in several groups.

Painkillers

These drugs (also known as analgesics) improve the comfort of the patient, but do nothing to treat the disease. Pain can be caused by injury, operation or disease, such as heart attack, cancer or pleurisy.

Painkillers commonly used are:

morphine	pethidine
codeine	fentanyl
alfentanil	sufentanil

An effect of these potent painkillers can be to reduce the desire to breathe and cough. Although most of the time this is an undesirable side-effect it can be useful if the patient is on a ventilator. The painkiller can also make the tube inserted into the windpipe (trachea) more tolerable.

Sedatives

An intensive care unit can be a frightening place for a patient. They can become very anxious at being linked to a confusing array of machines. The unit is also brightly lit and can be very noisy all day and night. Sometimes the noise level can be as loud as a bus passing close by (90 decibels). That makes getting rest difficult. To enable the patient to rest and reduce their anxiety sedatives are given. Some of these may only be given at night. Drugs commonly used in the group are:

midazolam	flunitrazepan
propofol	chlormethiazole
droperidol	haloperidol
diazepam (Valium®)	nitrazepam (Mogadon®)

Anaesthetic gases, such as isoflurane, may also be given through the ventilator into the breathing mix for this purpose.

Drugs for heart disease

Patients may already have a heart problem when they come to the ICU and need drugs to continue the treatment, or they may be given drugs on arrival in the ICU for a heart problem associated with their condition. Most of these drugs make the heart beat at a slower pace. Drugs that treat irregularities of the heart (arrhythmias) include:

digoxin	amiodarone
adenosine	lignocaine
verapramil	propranolol

There are some drugs that increase the heart rate such as:

atropine	adrenaline
isoprenaline	ephedrine

Other drugs act on the heart and blood vessels. When a patient suffers shock (Chapter 4) the heart and blood vessels can be affected. It may be necessary to use drugs to increase the force at which the heart pumps and to increase, or reduce, the diameter of the blood vessels. The drugs which increase the force at which the heart pumps are called inotropes. The drugs that widen the blood vessels – cause them to dilate – are called vasodilators. The drugs that narrow the blood vessels – cause them to constrict – are called vasoconstrictors.

Inotropes

These drugs that increase the power of each heart beat are useful in treating hearts that are affected by infection (Chapter 4, Shock), heart attacks, heart operations, or other heart injuries.

These drugs include:

adrenaline	dobutamine
dopexamine	dopamine

Vasoconstrictors

The blood vessels may be dilated by infection (sepsis) or a life-threatening allergic reaction to a drug or other substance. The heart can be working well but because blood vessels are wide there is little pressure in them. It is a bit like having a hose pipe with a wide opening at the end and the tap full on. Despite the large flow the water dribbles out. Some organs need high blood pressure to make them work properly, like the kidneys. A vasoconstrictor drug will make the blood vessels contract and reduce the diameter, thus raising the blood pressure.

Drugs most commonly used to make the blood vessels constrict (or reduce in diameter) are:

noradrenaline	dopamine
ephedrine	phenylephrine

Vasodilators

In some situations the blood vessels are constricted too much and need to be dilated. This usually happens when the heart is not pumping well. This is seen during severe blood loss and after heart attack (myocardial infarction). It can also happen in sepsis and during a severe allergic reaction to drugs or other substances.

If blood or fluid has been lost it must be replaced before the blood vessels are widened by a vasodilator drug or else there will be a dramatic drop in blood pressure. Vasodilator drugs are needed because the problem with constricted blood vessels is that they increase the workload of the heart. In most cases the heart finds it difficult to cope with the extra work. Vasodilator drugs most commonly used are:

dopexamine	dobutamine
sodium nitroprusside	glycerytrinitrate
	enoximone

Muscle relaxants

This is a group of drugs that paralyse all the voluntary muscles in the body, but not the involuntary muscles of the heart, gut, and bladder. Voluntary muscles are those you can choose to move and the muscles that control breathing. In some circumstances it can be necessary to temporarily paralyse these muscles. A small number of patients will need muscle relaxants when they are connected to a ventilator. In some cases the machine has to be able to override the normal breathing pattern. It can be dangerous for other patients on a ventilator to cough and strain, so a muscle relaxant will be given to stop coughing.

Being paralysed in this way, while still conscious, can be terrifying. For this reason all patients on relaxants are rendered unconscious and pain-free by giving them sedatives and painkillers.

This group of drugs includes:

suxamethonium	atracurium
rocuronium	pancuronium
vecuronium	mivacurium

Ulcer-preventing drugs

Being in an intensive care unit is sometimes stressful and this alone can cause ulcers. Ulcers are also a common problem with patients on ventilators, suffering from head injuries, and with kidney or liver failure. Patients in an intensive care unit are usually given ulcer-preventing drugs to reduce the acid secretion of the stomach as a preventative measure. These drugs are ranitidine and cimetidine, and are given as tablets, or intravenously. Another ulcer-preventing drug, that works by lining the stomach, is sucralfate. This is given through a nasogastric tube or as tablets. Some drugs may be stopped when nasogastric feeding starts.

Anti-diarrhoeal drugs

Diarrhoea is also a common problem in the critically ill because of a combination of factors. These can include antibiotics, nasogastric feeding which is an unnatural method of feeding, or infection present in the gut.

They can all cause irritation to the digestive system. Drugs commonly used to combat this problem are loperamide, codeine phosphate, and kaolin. All are given by nasogastric tube.

Laxatives

On the other side of the coin, constipation is quite a common problem with the seriously ill. It is one of the side-effects of painkillers, especially those which are morphine-based. The drug used in this case is lactulose.

Diuretics

Critically ill patients can end up with an excess of salt water inside their bodies. This is usually because too much fluid is contained in the feeding material entering the body via the gastric tube or intravenously. As part of the patient's illness or condition, tissues in the body may swell and fill with fluid. As the patient recovers these fluids and salts return to the circulation. Help has to be given to the patient to remove the unwanted fluids and salt from the body.

The critically ill patient may also have kidneys that are not working properly and this inevitably results in fluid retention. Sometimes it is also necessary to 'dry out' organs such as the lungs or brain if they become swollen. The drugs commonly used to remove unwanted fluids and salt from the body are:

frusemide   bumetamide
dopamine   dopexamine

All these drugs work on the kidneys and are infused into the body through a 'drip'.

Another drug quite commonly used is mannitol which is also fed through a drip. The effect of this drug is to make the urine more concentrated so the body adds more fluid to dilute it and so removing further fluid from the body.

Bronchodilators

Patients suffering from chest infections, or asthma may need bronchodilators. Their condition causes muscles in the tubes (bronchi) leading to the lungs to tighten. When this happens the airflow is reduced and it causes wheezing. Drugs are given to relax these muscles. These drugs are given into the veins or can be given directly to the lungs by inhaling them (nebulization). The drugs commonly used are salbutamol, which can be given intravenously or inhaled, and ipratropium, which is inhaled. Aminophylline can also be given but intravenously only.

Immunosuppressants

These, as the name suggests, suppress the body's natural immune system. These are most commonly used in organ transplants where it is necessary to stop the body rejecting the foreign organ that has been swapped from a donor into the patient's body.

Immunosuppressants are also needed if there has been some sort of allergic reaction by the body to itself so that the body's own immune system starts attacking organs and other parts of the body. The most commonly used immunosuppressants are:

hydrocortisone	prednisolone
cyclosporin	FK506

Antimicrobials

Infections can be caused by bacteria, fungi, and viruses. For bacteria we use antibiotics. For fungal infections antifungal drugs are used and for viral infections, specific antiviral agents are administered. Antimicrobial drugs will not deal with a major infection source by themselves and sometimes it needs a surgeon or a radiologist to drain an infected area or site of pus.

Antibiotics

These drugs need to be used in short bursts, up to seven days at a time, for various reasons. The most common reason is bacteria can build up a resistance to the antibiotics and also that antibiotics can be toxic. It is also not generally realized what a wide range of antibiotics the doctors have available to them. There are 80 major antibiotics in common use and each is targeted at a particular group of infections. Some infections are quite easily dealt with but others are resistant to attack by antibiotics and very difficult to deal with (Chapter 4, Shock).

The vast range of antibiotics in use in intensive care units include the famous penicillin family including ampicillin and flucloxacillin. Other families include the cephalosporins (cefotaxime, ceftazidime) and aminoglycosides (gentamicin, vancomycin). Metronidazole is useful against some sorts of organisms that don't need much oxygen as may cause abdominal infections

Antifungal agents

There is a much smaller range of antifungal agents. The most common site for fungal infections are the mouth, the groin, and the vaginal areas. Two well-known and common fungal infections are thrush and athlete's foot. In any seriously ill patient fungal infection can occur deep in any organ in the body. Transplant patients are at special risk from fungal infections because their natural defences have been suppressed to stop rejection of the transplanted organ.

An antifungal agent, which may be painted on the affected site, is nystatin. Others given intravenously are amphotericin and fluconazole.

Antiviral drugs

A patient being admitted to an intensive care unit can already be suffering from a viral infection or a virus can complicate the condition that caused the patient to arrive in the unit. Again, transplant patients are particularly susceptible to viral infections because their natural immune system has been suppressed to prevent organ rejection. There is a very limited range of anti-viral drugs available. If there were a full range we would by now have a cure for the common cold. The anti-viral drugs commonly used in intensive care are acyclovir and gancyclovir.

Hormones

Hormones are sometimes needed to regulate parts of the body. For example, diabetics need to regulate their doses of the hormone insulin and people who have damaged their pancreas become diabetic and also need insulin. Sometimes patients who are not diabetic become resistant to insulin as a reaction to stress and need infusions of this hormone. Insulin enables glucose to get from the blood to the living cells in the body so that it can be used as an energy source.

Steroids

Artificial steroids may sometimes be of benefit to patients in intensive care although they may have some unpleasant side-effects. There are many different sorts of steroids. The steroids used for critically ill patients are given to top-up the body's own natural levels which may help the seriously ill patient cope with stress. They are helpful in the reduction of some types of tissue swelling in the brain and in the lining of the bronchial tubes in asthma. Steroids are also used for immunosuppression, for example to prevent rejection of transplanted organs. Natural steroids are made in the adrenal glands which sit on top of the kidneys. The most common steroids administered are hydrocortisone and prednisolone.

Vitamins and minerals

All seriously ill patients need more vitamins and minerals than healthy people because there is an increased turnover of tissues within the body as damaged tissue is repaired.

People can also arrive in the intensive care unit with a vitamin deficiency because of their disease. We can only measure the effect of deficiency of one vitamin, vitamin K, which is essential for blood clotting. This can be discovered by laboratory tests because it is difficult to measure the effects, too much or too little may be given.

If too much of water-soluble vitamins are given they pass safely out of the body. Other vitamins can only be dissolved in fat and are given in carefully controlled amounts. Fat soluble vitamins can accumulate in the body and become poisonous. The vitamins most commonly given to ICU patients are B_{12}, folinic acid, and vitamin K. There are also multivitamin preparations given to patients.

Trace elements – such as copper, zinc, magnesium, and cobalt – are given in extremely small amounts.

Local anaesthetics

Just as at the dentist's, where local anaesthetic is given to kill the pain in one particular tooth, so anaesthetic drugs can be used in the intensive care unit to anaesthetize a particular part of the body.

The special skills of an anaesthetist will be needed as the site is quite often a few millimetres wide and deep within the body. The site can only be located by an experienced 'hand' feeling for the spot. Local anaesthetics commonly used in ICU are lignocaine and bupivacaine.

16

Feeding

Food and water are even more important for the critically ill patient receiving intensive care than for normal, fit and active people. It is not always appreciated that a sick or injured patient needs even more calories each day than a hard-working labourer. A working man requires about 8500 kiloJoules (2000 calories) per day to provide the energy to keep his lungs and heart working, provide the power for his muscles, and replenish the cells that are constantly recycled within the body. An intensive care patient can require one-and-a-half times that amount, up to 12 500 kiloJoules (3000 calories) a day. The body fighting for life needs that additional food to repair organs, bones or tissue injured by accident, disease or medical operations.

A healthy person can only function without water for up to three days. The body contains 40–50 litres of fluid and loses one-and-a-half litres through sweat and urine every 24 hours. Even fit young men die in 60 days without food. First the muscles start breaking down in a desperate bid to supply the missing nutritional material. Then the vital organs start shutting down to leave meagre supplies of food for the heart and brain. Critically ill patients, with greater demands on their bodies, would die much faster.

Wherever possible a patient, however ill, will be fed normally. Even plain, simple, natural food passing through the normal digestive system is far better than the most advanced artificial forms of nutrition.

Nursing staff will endeavour to spoon-feed patients with puréed or liquidized food, or give nutritionally complete drinks known as 'sip feeds', rather than introduce liquids and artificial foods into the body through tubes. Unfortunately critically ill patients frequently do need to be fed artificially, if only for short periods.

Artificial nutrition in various liquid forms still have to provide a balanced diet containing the essential protein, carbohydrates, fats, vitamins, and trace elements normally derived from our traditional 'three square meals'. Protein is often given already broken down into its building blocks of amino acids to help rapid absorption into the body. Artificial feeding, like all aspects of intensive care, has developed into a sophisticated science. Each cocktail of essential foods is mixed with the aid of dieticians to match the individual requirements of each patient.

These artificial foods have to be 'fed' to the patient who cannot eat or drink. This is done in one of four ways, all using a tube. The tube can be inserted through the nose straight into the digestive system (enteral feeding) or intravenously by placing it into a vein in the chest (parenteral feeding).

We will simply describe each in turn:

- **Nasogastric feeding**. A tube is passed through the nose, down through the throat, and into the stomach.

- **Nasojejunal feeding** The tube also passes through the stomach and into the small bowel.

- **Gastrostomy** or **jejujostomy**. The stomach is a reservoir for food and, in the critically ill patient, drugs and other substances. These drugs may cause the stomach to stop working. Injury or infection, or a combination of these, can also prevent feeding through the stomach by causing it to stop functioning. When it is not possible to place a tube into the nose, either because of injury or surgery, then it is possible to insert the tube straight into the stomach or small bowel with a minor operation. This is often used to feed people with long-term problems with feeding.

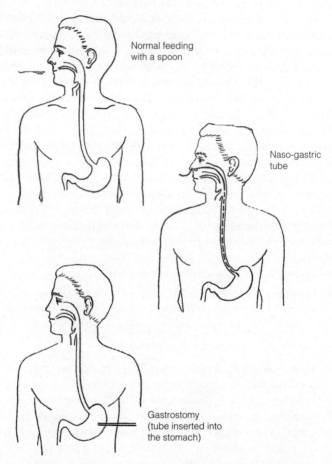

Normal feeding
with a spoon

Naso-gastric
tube

Gastrostomy
(tube inserted into
the stomach)

Different positions of tubes for feeding into the stomach.

Both these methods of passing artificial food into the lower digestive system can have problems. It is a very unnatural way to receive food. A side-effect can be violent diarrhoea. The food has to be adjusted to compensate for these complications and frequently additives such as the well-known kaolin and morphine have to be introduced into the food to correct this problem. The food is contained in one bag or bottle and fed almost continuously.

Feeding problems are increased when the normal digestive system is not working for some reason. It is then necessary to introduce the vital nutritional fluid straight into the blood supply, that is intravenously.

There are two types of intravenous feeding. Peripheral vein feeding involves inserting the tube into a small vein, either on the back of the hand or elsewhere on the arm. Full intravenous feeding involves inserting a larger tube into a large vein in the chest near the heart.

Using a small vein causes difficulties. The essential salts and other chemicals contained in the artificial food cocktail can cause a great deal of irritation to the delicate vein so the food solution has to be very diluted. To adequately feed a critically ill patient through a small vein it would require between 4–6 litres – that's 8–12 pints – of this feed each day. It is just not possible to pass that volume of fluid into a body already having other lifesaving fluids pumped into it. This form of intravenous feeding has to be reserved for occasions when other forms of feeding are impractical.

Full intravenous feeding, using a larger vein in the chest, allows the amount of fluid with the food to be reduced to about 2.5 litres. This is because there is a greater flow of blood passing the catheter which helps to dilute the irritating material, but this method does have increased risks. The doctor inserting the tube has to be particularly careful not to damage vital organs such as the lungs or arteries in this area of the chest. There are also greater risks of infection.

With both intravenous methods the amino acids, carbo-hydrates, fats, and other ingredients to the food cocktail are often contained in separate bottles leading eventually to the one tube. Infusion pumps (Chapter 13, Equipment) accu-rately measure and control prescribed quantities of each ingredient. These can then be varied according to the patient's individual requirements.

Visitors will notice that in some ICUs bottles may have a bright coloured tab which can be green, amber, or red, cor-responding to the colour on the tap controlling its supply. Medical and nursing staff refer to these taps as the 'traffic lights' because of their colour. The colours just make it easy to see which tap controls the supply from which bottle.

All these intravenous feeding methods require food to be introduced constantly, around the clock, and not at set meal times. Once a patient's feeding requirements are stable it is possible for all the ingredients to be mixed in one 'big bag' as it is known and fed through one simple control.

17

Feelings

'Can they hear me?' That's one of the first questions asked by relatives and visitors to unconscious patients in intensive care. The answer has to be 'We don't really know, but talk to them anyway, the staff will.' Talking to even deeply unconscious patients does at least remind everyone that they are an individual human being with feelings.

Some drugs given to render patients unconscious and relieve anxiety will block out memory absolutely so they will not remember you talking to them even if they had been able to hear you at the time. The best example is midazolam, a powerful amnesic. Patients who have been treated with this drug can rarely recall events that happened while they were receiving it, not even in dreams or nightmares that draw on the subconscious memory. Some patients recovering in intensive care dislike this loss of memory and the lack of control over their own destiny.

A common experience of patients recovering from severe disease and emerging from a drugs regime is a period of great agitation, worry and stress. Patients themselves may have no recollection of that time but it can cause relatives and visitors great concern. Some patients can also behave in a confused and delirious fashion. This is usually caused by withdrawal of drugs and sleep deprivation. Research has found that drug-induced sleep bears little resemblance to real sleep and it may not have the same benefits. The only similarity is that the eyes are closed.

Hallucinations are commonly reported including seeing snakes and even pink elephants! Perhaps the number of tubes surrounding the patients during recovery affects them and brings on these sightings. Many recovering patients have visions of people standing in front of them speaking to them and sometimes become confused by the reflection of nurses and visitors in windows and believe they are the real people. These are all common problems.

A lack of proper sleep contributes to this state. Many former ICU patients have recalled that their experience as they recovered was similar to that of being a terrorist hostage. They suffered a constant fear of imminent death, a great deal of discomfort, and a lack of sleep.

Drugs can relieve specific pains, but there is nothing that can dispel the general feeling of discomfort that patients in intensive care suffer. The unit is necessarily well lit, but staff do try to introduce a feeling of day and night by dimming lights or erecting curtains around patients at night to try and assist their sleep. Clocks can also help orientate patients as to the time of day but there can be disadvantages. Some patients tend to become clock watchers and this makes the day drag on endlessly for them.

Some ICUs, particularly in continental Europe, treat people fighting for life in separate rooms. This has several drawbacks for the staff. There is a need for more nurses to be on duty and those nurses feel isolated from each other. It can also be boring for the recovering patients who like to watch the activity going on around them in an open-plan ward.

Boredom can be one of the worst problems for patients in intensive care. It can add to the almost inevitable depression patients suffer to some degree. Severe depression can lead to demands from some seriously ill patients to have their life support removed. This is never done. These suicidal thoughts soon disappear when the patient recovers.

Television, videos, radio, music, talking books, letters, and cards all help relieve the monotony. Most of all patients welcome visitors. Many intensive care units have open visiting (throughout the 24 hours) although for practical reasons morning and late night visits are less welcome. Some do not allow visitors during ward rounds. Visitors should, of course, respect other patients' need for privacy and peace.

Visitors should also realize that there are occasions when their arrivals will be delayed by emergencies or other work on the unit. Similarly, visitors who realize there is a problem or crisis developing within the unit should use their common sense and slip away quietly.

Visitors to patients fighting for life naturally suffer a roller coaster of emotions from elation at signs of recovery to depression at any setback. These highs and lows will occur many times during recovery. These anxieties are extremely tiring. Visitors, particularly close relatives of long-stay patients, are well advised to try and maintain as normal a lifestyle as possible. They must continue to work if possible and maintain the usual pattern of sleeping, eating, and exercise.

Relatives should not feel obliged to spend the day at the bedside of the sick loved one. They should remember they will spend far more time visiting as the patient recovers. Their time and strength will be needed at this later stage. Advice may be needed about travelling a long distance to visit someone seriously ill and who has been recently admitted to an intensive care unit, or on such subjects as taking compassionate leave from work. This advice should always be sought from a senior member of staff, at least a consultant or senior registrar, not a junior nurse or junior member of the medical staff.

Relatives will also meet visitors to other ICU patients in the waiting room. It is only natural that there will be discussions between visitors about the care and treatment of their own loved ones. A great deal of this information exchange will be valuable. It is possible, however, that some information could be misleading and cause unnecessary worry. If you are concerned in any way about anything, please consult the nurse looking after the patient.

Visitors should always try to act as normally as possible when they arrive at the patient's bedside. If it is their normal practice to greet the person with a hug and kiss then they should carry on with that greeting if possible.

Children should also be offered the chance to visit. Young children tend not to take too much notice of the machinery and tubes surrounding the patient. They only see their mother, brother, uncle, etc. Often children's chatter and play can be a great comfort and they should be encouraged to bring their toys with them. It is also worth enquiring whether pets can visit. Old people benefit from seeing a much loved cat or dog. Blind people develop a very special relationship with their guide dogs and visits of these animals will be allowed if at all possible, but you must bear in mind that some more rare or exotic pets may be a problem, but do ask as it may be possible to overcome it.

What presents to bring the patient often causes a problem. Most intensive care units, except coronary care units, do not allow flowers because of the infection risk to other patients. Always welcome are books of short stories, magazines — particularly those with lots of pictures — holiday brochures, music tapes, or CDs. If the patient is eating normally, food is also a popular choice, although the type of food should be checked with staff beforehand. Strawberries, grapes, chocolates, and bananas can be poisonous, particularly to kidney patients, because they contain lots of potassium.

Grateful visitors and former patients often want to give something to staff on the unit. The nicest present is a thank-you letter and a Christmas card. Again, music tapes and CDs will give staff and patients hours of enjoyment. Money donated, however little, can be used towards buying important machinery which can often cost £20 000 or more. There are often local funds to promote intensive care research and the Intensive Care Society has its own fund for nationally organized research. All these organizations are always grateful for any donations.

Visitors sometimes notice that doctors and nurses rarely show any emotion in the intensive care unit. That does not mean that they do not suffer distress, grief, or sadness at the fate or plight of their patients. They do. They often have their own strategies to cope with the traumas of their work. One of the most popular is humour and often the jokes might shock visitors who overhear them. They should realize it is just a way for the staff to get rid of their own tensions and feelings.

The doctors and nurses also organize frequent social and sporting events for the same reason — to let off the steam that they can so rarely relieve at work. Their apparent coolness and efficiency does not mean they are unfeeling or callous. They *do* care when someone dies and you must remember that between 15% and 30% of the patients entering intensive care do not win their fight for life. But the staff still have to carry on working for the other patients battling to recover. Normal human relations do develop between doctors, nurses, and patients. It is not always possible for everyone to get on well with every patient. Difficult and cantankerous people do not necessarily change their personality when they become seriously ill and frustrations and frictions can arise. Doctors and nurses work extremely long hours and they also get tired like everyone else. This should always be remembered.

18

Dying

Patients entering an intensive care unit are literally fighting for their lives. Without intensive care many would die. But it is not a battle that every intensive care patient will win despite the combined efforts of the skilled nursing, medical, and technical staffs. The very advances that have enabled life to be saved in intensive care could also be used to delay death. A point may be reached when the patient's condition is so overwhelming there is nothing more that can be done for them. In these circumstances the medical team, after discussion with the relatives, may decide to let the patient – who will not survive – die with dignity. This can be done immediately by withdrawing treatment, that is switching off the life-preserving machines and apparatus, such as the ventilator. Death will occur but this is not euthanasia (which is illegal in the UK but allowed in a few parts of the world) as there is no outside assistance. Nature is simply allowed to take its course.

A common reason for treatment being withdrawn is brain death. A patient with suspected severe brain damage will be admitted to an intensive care unit and placed on a ventilator to keep their lungs working. The suspected damage may be the result of a head injury during an accident, a stroke, or the brain being starved of oxygen during drowning or suffocation. The patient has to be given a chance to recover but if there are no signs of brain activity then brain death may be established. All further life support or treatment will be futile. The concept of brain death, when the rest of the body appears to be working, was first recognized by two French doctors in 1959. They labelled it *le coma depassé*.

In Britain, surgeons, anaesthetists, and physicians have agreed a set of seven tests to establish brain death. These tests have to be carried out twice by two doctors — a total of four times. One of the doctors has to be a consultant, the other one can be either a senior registrar or another consultant. Before the tests can begin the doctors have to be satisfied that they know what caused brain death. They must make sure the patient's body is at the normal temperature otherwise the tests may be wrong. They must check there is no major abnormality in the body chemistry and must ensure that no drugs are still in the body that could effect the brain or muscles. The tests check each area of the brain in turn. A brain-scanning EEG (electroencephalogram) is not needed in Britain. Some other countries do use them to diagnose brain stem death.

The British tests are:

- a bright light does not cause the eyes to move
- touching the eyes does not cause a blink
- cold water squirted in the ears brings no reaction
- pain inflicted on the body causes no flinching or movement
- an object placed in the mouth does not cause 'gagging'
- touching the tube leading to the lungs (the trachea) does not cause coughing
- the patient cannot breathe without the aid of a machine.

Transplant surgery can also lead to a situation where treatment in an intensive care unit may be withdrawn. As part of the so-called 'swap-op' drugs are used to suppress the body's immune system to prevent the transplanted organ (heart, kidney, or liver) being rejected. An infection may

occur which the body cannot fight because its normal
defences have been put out of action. The doctors in intensive care will find themselves in a 'no-win' predicament —
treat the infection and the organ will be rejected and the
patient will die — leave the infection to take its course and
the patient will die. In these circumstances a decision may
well be taken to withdraw life support.

Life and death decisions are difficult for all concerned.
Perhaps the most difficult is where some doubt may exist
that death is inevitable. In this case a decision may be made
to withdraw a specific treatment if a patient's condition
deteriorates to a point where death will result. This could
happen, for example, with a patient still dying from cancer,
despite a major operation, who then develops other infections and complications. It may be possible to keep this
patient living for a time until the cancer eventually kills
them. A decision could be taken that if vital organs
attacked by these other infections stop working, no effort
will be made to artificially start them again. This is known
as a 'Do Not Escalate' order and is a much debated and
controversial subject. In some cases, particularly with
cancer patients, it may be possible to consult the patient
about how far they want to continue their fight for life and
agree at what stage no further efforts will be made to save
them. The death certificate will contain the eventual cause
of death and possibly the original condition that brought
the patient to intensive care. If the cause of death was an
accident, deliberate act, or death occurred in suspicious circumstances the Coroner has to be informed by law. He
may then decide to have a post-mortem and hold an
inquest. The doctors have no say in these matters. A
coroner's officer, usually a serving police officer, will then
have to interview and take statements from witnesses to
the original action that brought the patient to intensive
care, and relatives and medical staff. If an inquest is held,
once the coroner has heard all the evidence, he or she will

record a verdict which will state the cause of death. This could be 'accidental death', 'misadventure', or 'death by natural causes'.

In Britain the situations when death must be reported to the Coroner are listed below:

- The body is unidentified
- No doctor attended the patient in the last 14 days of life
- Death occurred during operation or recovery from anaesthesia
- Any sudden or unexplained death
- Medical mishaps
- Death related to an industrial accident or disease
- Death following violence, neglect, abortion, accident, or misadventure
- Death occurring in suspicious or unnatural circumstances
- Alcoholism
- Poisoning
- Prisoners (including those in Police custody)
- Pensioners (service disability)

19

Organ donation

For the past 25 years it has been possible for organs to be transplanted from one person to another. This started with kidneys and corneas (which form part of the eye). Now the list has grown to include the heart, heart valves, lungs, liver, pancreas, small bowel, skin, and bones.

Organs from one person can save the lives of several others in a series of 'swop-ops'. The donor has two kidneys, and so two patients suffering kidney failure can receive one each. Even if a donor's death is caused by damage to one or more vital organs, those unaffected may still be suitable for transplant.

There are 1500 people each year in Britain who are pronounced brain dead after admission to intensive care units who would make suitable organ donors. Tests to establish brain-stem death are carried out twice by two doctors (Chapter 18, Dying). Permission for organ donation, if not already given, is usually sought after brain death has been provisionally diagnosed by the first set of tests and before the final series is carried out. There is usually from 3–24 hours between the two sets of tests. This can be used to give transplant teams time to prepare and time for the families to consider the request if necessary. Only after the final set of tests confirm brain death will the patient be taken to an operating theatre for organs to be removed.

Patients dying in intensive care will be considered as organ donors if there has been a wish expressed by the patient to donate organs or relatives think the patient would have wished to be an organ donor. If a patient becomes hopelessly ill and is obviously dying then relatives may wish to consult doctors about organ donation. It is necessary for doctors to be made aware of the patient's or relatives' wishes *before* death occurs so that transplant operations can be organized and coordinated. The people waiting to receive vital organs may be a considerable distance away, perhaps even in another country.

Organs perish at different rates once the heart stops and the supply of oxygen and nutrients is stopped. The heart, lungs, liver, pancreas, and small bowel can survive for only a matter of minutes after death. The kidneys are damaged after about four hours and the corneas within 24 hours.

Although the brain is dead there are still natural reflexes that exist as a result of nerve action controlled by the spinal cord and not the brain. The heart and lungs continue to work. Drugs are given to stop these reflex movements and changes in heart rate and blood pressure. There is still a small minority of doctors who do not believe in the concept of brain-stem death and only believe life is extinct when the heart stops beating naturally.

Although many people in Britain carry organ donor cards there are times when their wishes may be overruled. If an inquest is required into the patient's death then the Coroner or Procurator Fiscal (in Scotland) may stop transplant plans because he wants various organs preserved or examined – especially if some court action is involved. Technically if someone dies in hospital then the body belongs to the hospital and relatives have no legal power. The hospital may have some reason for stopping some organ donation. It is, however, usual for relatives to be fully consulted and their wishes taken into account.

In Britain we have a system where potential organ donors 'opt in' to the transplant scheme through donor cards or registering their desire to donate organs in some other way. Many other countries have a 'opt out' system. This means organs will be taken for transplant unless the potential donor has registered a desire for their body not to be used for transplantation. It is unknown whether introducing the 'opt out' system in Britain would increase the number of donated organs. The Intensive Care Society has advocated there should be no change in our system unless there is a proven benefit to the donor organ supply.

Intensive care does not stop and the patient is not treated as a potential organ donor until death is certified after the second set of brain death tests.

There are a number of reasons why organs may not be used for transplanting. These contraindications may be the presence of diseases in the donor, such as AIDS, or hepatitis B, which could be passed on to the recipient. There may also be damage to the organs being considered for donation. This can be from injury or disease, such as diabetes. It may simply be that the organs have been worn out through old age. There may also be problems finding a suitable recipient who shares the donor's blood group and tissue type. Specially trained transplant coordinators are always available when organ donation is being considered. They coordinate between all members of the medical profession involved and the relatives. They help organize the retrieval of donor organs and the various transplant operations. No details of the people who receive the organs are disclosed and relatives of donors are urged not to try and find out their identities.

It is important to realize that one body used for organ donation can relieve the suffering of eight or more people. Many relatives of people whose organs are used for transplants feel that some good has come from tragedy and their relative did not die in vain.

In Britain the UK Transplant Service (based in Bristol) assists in the matching of donors to recipients. Elsewhere in Europe, Eurotransplant and Scand Transplant carry out the same work. There is an organization in Britain, called BODY, that helps people come to terms with the trauma associated with organ donation. Its address is care of Mr Evans, BODY, Balsham, Cambridge, CB 16DL.

20

Research

Intensive care is a new area of medicine that has developed over the last 35 years. Many of the techniques and new drugs used in intensive care have not been subjected to controlled trials to see if they actually work as intended. New treatments are usually better but sometimes something unexpected can happen which will make the new drug or treatment *less* effective than an old 'tried and tested' one.

New drugs that may benefit the critically ill have to be tested at some stage on those very people – the critically ill. It is more ethical to use volunteers among intensive care patients to carry out that essential research rather than to introduce the drug untried among all seriously ill people who may, or may not, benefit from it. A new drug or technique can seem miraculous in theory, but because the seriously ill don't react to drugs in the normal predicted way good ideas can be bad medicine.

Doctors trying to advance medical knowledge and improve the care of the critically ill do need to carry out tests and experiments with volunteers. It is important to remember that such trials are extremely carefully controlled and monitored. The proposed study of a new drug or technique is based on extensive knowledge of the benefits to other patients. A detailed plan of the proposed experiment is written. This then has to be approved by an

Ethical Committee before it can start. That Committee's job is to protect the patient from any study that may contain any unnecessary or excessive risk. They also ensure that adequate information is given to the patient and/or relatives and friends so they can make an informed decision about whether or not to take part in such a trial.

It must be emphasized that taking part in such research is entirely voluntary. Any patient not wishing to take part in a study will not jeopardize their care in any way.

All research is guided by the Declaration of Helsinki 1964, regularly amended and published by the World Medical Association. This declaration is designed to stop patients being exploited in any way and to ensure the information gained is really medically useful.

Before any research can start written consent is usually obtained from the patient or the next of kin. All research is carefully scrutinized as it progresses. Some experiments are even visited by international monitoring organizations randomly to ensure they are properly conducted.

Some patients and their families may find the decision as to whether to take part in any research or experiment very distressing. They realize a new drug could be useful but are worried about possible dangers. They should always ask for time to consider their decision.

There are occasions when a new drug, or an apparent breakthrough in medical science, is suddenly given to an individual patient. This is not research but usually a 'last-ditch' attempt to save life. This happened with a revolutionary Japanese drug FK506. It was developed to prevent rejection of transplanted organs. It was flown to Britain to save the life of a patient despite no research into its benefits being carried out in this country. Since then that research has been carried out in proper trials and its place in the catalogue of available drugs realized.

A part of the trials of new drugs may involve the use of placebos. A placebo is a substance that closely resembles the drug in appearance but has no effect whatsoever. Placebos are given to some of the patients taking part in the research, and neither the doctors nor the patients know who is given the drug and who is given the placebo until the trial is completed. The idea is to ensure that the research is not influenced by the doctors running the study or the power of the patient's own mind. It has been found in the past that patients believing they are receiving a new wonder drug have shown a remarkable improvement in their condition even though they have only been receiving water. The mind is a powerful aid to recovery.

All research is submitted for publication so that all the medical profession can benefit from the results. Individual patients taking part in any experiment or research are never identified in these reports.

Common abbreviations

AIDS	Acquired immune deficiency syndrome
ALT	alanie aminotransferase
ARDS	acute respiratory distress syndrome
ASB	assisted spontaneous breathing
CMV	continuous mandatory ventilation
CPAP	constant positive airway pressure
CT	computerized tomography (sometimes known as CAT)
CVP	central venous pressure
ECG	electrocardiogram
EEG	electroencephalogram
FFP	fresh frozen plasma
ICU	intensive care unit
IPPV	intermittent positive pressure ventilation
ITU	intensive therapy unit, another name for the ICU
kPa	kiloPascals (similar but different in size to mmHg)
mmHg	millimetres of mercury
$PaCO_2$	amount of carbon dioxide in the blood
PaO_2	amount of oxygen in the blood
PEEP	positive end expiratory pressure
PICU	paediatric intensive care unit
SpO_2	oxygen saturation in the blood
SIMV	synchronized intermittent ventilation
SCBU	special care baby unit (pronounced 'skibboo')

Index

In the index we have deliberately used medical terms and commonly used abbreviations, rather than the lay term. We felt that this would allow the reader hearing a term they didn't understand to find easily the explanation.

Index